仁神術

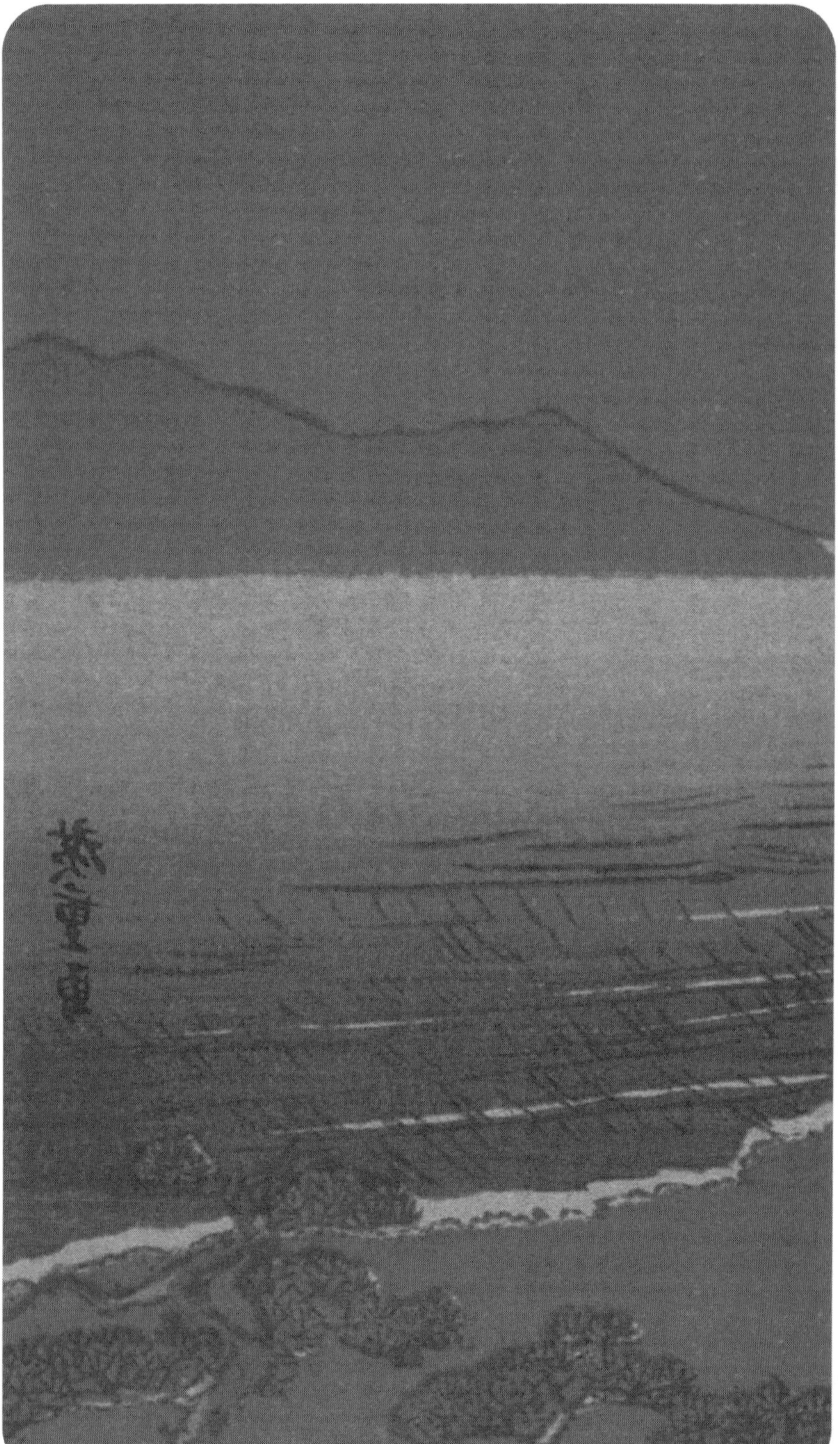

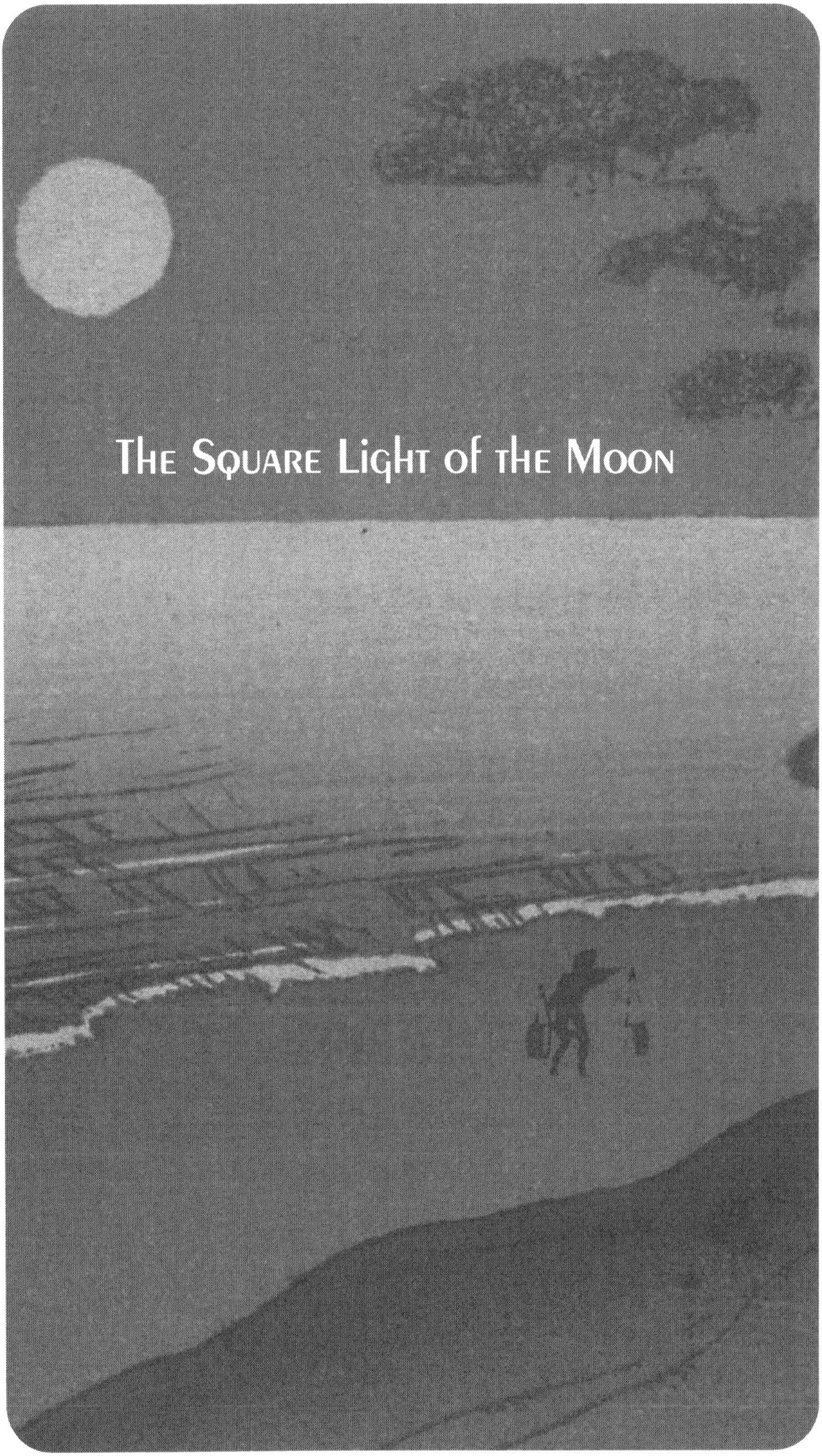
The Square Light of the Moon

茗

The Square Light of the Moon

A Journey of Healing with Jin Shin Jyutsu

∞

an Ancestral Japanese Medicine

Véronique Le Normand

Translated from the French
by Christiane Guillois

Upper West Side Philosophers, Inc.

New York

Published by Upper West Side Philosophers, Inc., New York, NY 10025, USA / www.westside-philosophers.com / www.yogaforthemind.us

Upper West Side Philosophers, Inc. provides a publication venue for original philosophical thinking steeped in lived life, in line with our motto: philosophical living & lived philosophy.

Cover Image: Anonymous Japanese woodcut, "A Fairy Moon and a Lonely Shore" (1890 – LCCN2008680225 / LoC ID: jpd.01557)
Design: Anne-Laure Exbrayat, Studio Graphique Actes Sud & UWSP, Inc.

Library of Congress Cataloging-in-Publication Data

Names: Le Normand, Véronique, 1955- author. | Guillois, Christiane, translator.
Title: The square light of the moon : a journey of healing with jin shin jyutsu : an ancestral Japanese medicine / Véronique Le Normand ; translated from the French by Christiane Guillois.
Other titles: Lumière carrée de la lune. English.
Description: New York : Upper West Side Philosophers, Inc., [2021] | Translation of: La lumière carrée de la lune : Jin Shin Jyutsu, une médecine ancestrale japonaise. | Includes bibliographical references. |
Summary: "Véronique Le Normand is a journalist and writer residing in Paris. In 2002, in the wake of a traumatic experience of loss, a doctor introduced her to Jin Shin Jyutsu, a Japanese art of healing that teaches us how to help ourselves simply through the use of our hands. In 2017, after fifteen years of study and practice, she set off for Japan to learn about the healer and samurai Jiro Murai, who had revived this physio-philosophy at the beginning of the twentieth century. Accompanied by her friend Kyoko Watanabe, Véronique retraced the steps of the elusive master, accompanied in spirit by the presence of seventeenth-century Japanese poet Basho. "The Square Light of the Moon" is the journal of a journey from one shore to another, and a marvelous initiation into Japanese culture"-- Provided by publisher.
Identifiers: LCCN 2020051286 | ISBN 9781935830719 (trade paperback) | ISBN 9781935830726 (epub)
Subjects: LCSH: Le Normand, Véronique, 1955---Health. | Acupressure--Japan. | Traditional medicine--Japan.
Classification: LCC RM723.A27 N676 2021 | DDC 615.8/2220952--dc23
LC record available at https://lccn.loc.gov/2020051286

For my dearest Kyoko
in memory of her beloved mother,
the writer Yoko Mochizuki,
whose name means
"full moon"

For all my loved ones

On his return from the land of Yomi, the land of death and defilement, the deity Izanagi threw off his clothes, giving birth to Yaso magatsuhi no kami and Oho magatsuhi no kami, deities of misfortune and calamity, who were immediately countered by Kamu nahobi no kami and Oho nahobi no kami, deities of remedy and healing.

– Records of Ancient Matters[1]

Contents

Should the wind be mighty
And carry you off
With the clouds
As far away as the Great Harmony
Your memory will remain with me still.

– *Kojiki*[2]

I

How Jin Shin Jyutsu Came Into My Life

Out of the Blue
A Big Cairn
A Gift

In the beginning was a tragedy.

September 2002.

I was outside my house in the Vercors region of France when the call came. It was to upend my life completely. I was gardening when the phone rang.

My brother had collapsed.

My younger brother lay on the floor, lifeless.

Felled by a ruptured aneurysm.

Thierry was a master glassblower. He had been working in his workshop, in Brittany. One minute he was standing at his workbench, the next he had fallen to the floor in a crash of shattered glass. They found him a few hours later. The radio was still on. Only a week before we had been together in this very garden in the mountains. With the help of his two boys, Victor and Rémi, he had built a limestone cairn, a big one taller than all of us and crowned with a rusted piece of iron twisted into the shape of a cross, and which birds perched on.

The period of mourning began.

My brother and I were only two years apart. My childhood memories washed away with my tears, my adolescent dreams lay crushed beneath surges of anger. I had lost a part of myself.

I no longer knew who I was in my own family.

I found myself drifting in a formless world.

Between the visible and the invisible.

It was as if I were in some Japanese film, like Kiyoshi Kurosawa's *Journey to the Shore* or Kenji Mizoguchi's *Tales of Ugetsu*.

In October, my friend Danielle, who the year before had lost her only child, Mathilde, took me to Avignon to see the doctor who had helped her. During his hour-long sessions, he would put his hands on various places of a patient's body. Twice I underwent this treatment without asking questions. Twice I left his office feeling at peace, or at least more at peace. The third time I confided to him my fears about a mammogram I was to have in two weeks. The radiologist had noticed a troubling spot. What the doctor prescribed was most peculiar: "We are going to determine together a moment of the day when you can be alone. During that time you will hold your index finger for fifteen minutes and focus on your breathing. You will do that every day until your appointment."

Hold my index finger!

I laughed, but I did it.

I had not laughed in weeks. Every day, I held my index finger. Every day I laughed to myself. I laughed thinking of the doctor who had prescribed this exercise. I pictured myself doing this and I laughed at this woman alleviating the sufferings of life by holding her index finger. I laughed imagining the look on the faces of people to whom it would be better not to mention this. I laughed when I thought of my brother, imagining him, too, howling with laughter. Two weeks later, it was the radiologist who was laughing as she informed me that my breast was fine. Was it then that I realized that the Buddha is always represented smiling?

It was April 2003.

I was unaware of it, but I had just engaged in my first self-help exercise in Jin Shin Jyutsu.

At the end of May, the good doctor came up to Paris. He was in need of office space. I let him use my study in exchange for which he treated my niece.

Mélanie was depressed. After just one session with him she began to climb out of the hole she was in.

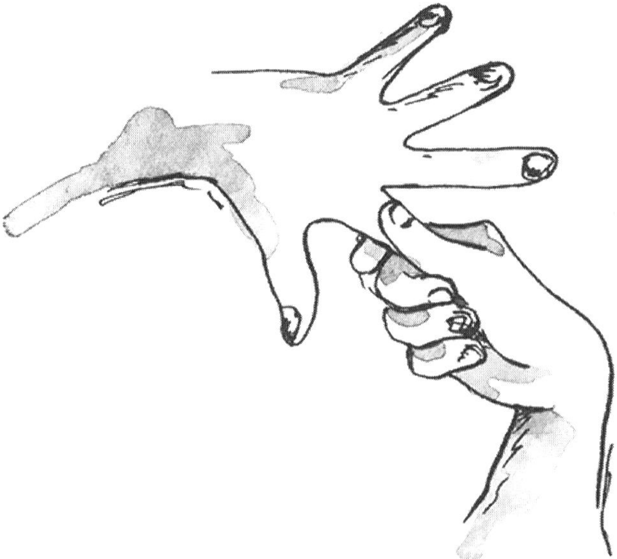

Holding one's index finger to fight fear.

The journalist in me also resurfaced: "Doesn't this tire you out? Where did you learn this practice? Is it a gift? If so, how did you come to know you had it?"

Patrick Nasica very calmly replied, "What I do, you can do, too."

Me? Do what? I can heal myself?

I had a substantial medical history that dated back to my childhood. I had seen many doctors, swallowed a multitude of pills, had numerous operations...

Be my own caregiver?

My younger brother had died unexpectedly. It seemed logical that I was next in line.

Help others?

Everyone in our family was suffering. There was plenty of work to be done.

Days passed and my sadness remained. There seemed no way out. But suddenly, after that one session of Jin Shin Jyutsu, I had felt lighter. My appetite returned and I found myself joking with friends and family. I began gardening and writing again. Something had changed. "What I do, you can do, too." His words resonated in me with the promise of comfort. By simply holding a finger you could initiate change and move from one state to another. It was so very simple, and it was accessible every moment of every day and required no medication and had no side effects. The simplicity of it made it seem almost supernatural. Surely the person who had said "hold your index finger" had access to some secret of nature. He was offering to share it with me. I wanted to know more. I wanted to know everything. My curiosity was growing by the hour.

A few days later, I knocked on the door of the French Jin Shin Jyutsu Association. As in Japan, I removed my shoes and, barefoot, stepped onto Natalie Max's tatami. The practitioner simply explained that Jin Shin Jyutsu had originated in Japan and that it was an art that involved harmonizing energies. It was taught in five-day seminars, and there were also shorter workshops that focused on self-help practices. Jin Shin Jyutsu was about "learning to know ourselves," which is something we never stop doing.

What I remember most from our conversation that first day was that Jin Shin Jyutsu, which I could not even pronounce, was the work of a man named Jiro Murai who had been born into a long line of doctors in Japan at the end of the 19th century but who chose to follow a path of his own. Then he took critically ill. At twenty-six, knowing his illness was terminal, he asked to be taken to the mountains to die. There he meditated, fasted, and performed mudras. One week later, to everyone's astonishment, he walked out of his retreat totally cured. He decided to dedicate the remainder of his life to studying this art of healing he named Jin Shin Jyutsu.

It was time for me to go back to the mountains in the Vercors and to the garden where I had received the news of my brother's death and where Thierry had erected his giant cairn. I could still see him carting stones in his wheelbarrow, carefully setting them in place to make sure they would hold, stepping back to examine his work. Thierry was a builder, and the cairn now embodied his person. I was impatient to get back to this symbol of his presence at my home.

The cairn had fallen down.

Undone by freezing temperatures.

The stones lay scattered on the ground. What was I supposed to do? Push them aside? Remove them from the garden?

I thought of a stone garden, like the ones they have in Japan. If the stones would not hold up vertically I could lay them out horizontally. I could arrange them in a circle that I would put where the cairn had stood. The thought absolutely delighted me. The cairn had not disappeared; its shape had simply changed. Today this stone garden casts its light on the surrounding vegetation like a large white moon. And when the fog settles in and I gaze upon that garden, I sometimes see my brother's cairn.

Of Nature
In a Single Breath
Hands

Jin Shin Jyutsu required nothing other than my hands, just the right one and the left. I had always thought mine small and not particularly attractive. They could not play the piano and could not draw very well, either. Yet Jiro Murai said that they were my greatest allies. That summer of 2003, I began to know my hands. Each one had five fingers, a palm, and a back. I could feel my heart beating in my index finger when I held it. When I closed my eyes I could feel fluid moving beneath my skin. I would focus on my breathing and feel the flow traveling through my body. I no longer felt totally lost; I had discovered a way to connect with myself. I was taking charge of myself. I realized that each finger was linked to a particular attitude towards life. By holding my index finger I could deal with fear. By holding my middle finger, with anger; my ring finger, sadness; my little finger, pretense; my thumb, worry. As a baby, I had ravenously sucked my thumb; had I really been that anxious? Whenever I was on a train or a bus, or watching a movie or television, I would hold one of my fingers, and an hour later I would feel the way you do when you come out of an *onsen*, a Japanese thermal bath: cleansed, purified, and at peace. I was elated to see that I could do this on my own. My brother's death had plummeted me into the void. Nature, which abhors a vacuum, had given me Jin Shin Jyutsu. If someone had told me that it took several years of study to learn this art, I would probably have looked elsewhere.

I was won over by the pleasure I derived from these sensations, which would come so suddenly. And there was nothing to learn, no physical effort to make, no equipment to get. Jin Shin Jyutsu suited me perfectly. Its exquisite simplicity was a source of joy. My fingers kept me company. Thierry and I had made clay castings of our hands. I kept one of them and still use it as a paperweight. We used to like to trace our hands and compare them: his, big, broad, and confident; mine, barely good enough to pray with. When we were students, he in the fine arts, I in literature, we loved to share things we came upon. Thierry introduced me to Albrecht Dürer and his studies of hands. He gave me a reprint of *Praying Hands*, a black ink and pencil drawing on blue paper that the artist had first called just *Hands*. I would turn to it all the time. In those hands lay all the love, gratitude, and compassion in the world. *Praying Hands* reminded me of the essential role that physical gestures play in all religions. To bring your palms together is to place yourself in a position in which to balance the relationship between body and soul.

Our family used to say that my brother had hands of gold. He painted, drew, sculpted stone, made stained-glass panels, and built his own house.

We had been raised in the Catholic religion. From the classes I had on the life of Jesus I retained that he was a healer and could perform miracles by placing his hands on a person. Jiro Murai said there was a healer in all of us. I knew nothing about Jin Shin Jyutsu, but I felt it to be beautiful, vast, just, and part of me.

The title of the first Jin Shin Jyutsu book I read was *Introducing Jin Shin Jyutsu Is*, its subtitle, *Getting to KNOW (Help) MYSELF, Art of Living*.[3]

Whenever I suddenly felt fatigued, I would sit on my hands.

When I had a headache, I would hold my head in my hands.

When I found it hard to breathe, I would place my hands on my elbows.

When I had problems digesting, I would put one hand on my cheek and the other on the collarbone on the same side.

When I was in need of comfort, I would hug myself, placing my hands under my armpits, and take thirty-six breaths.

"Be your own testimony," Jin Shin Jyutsu said. I practiced it, experimented with it, and felt better.

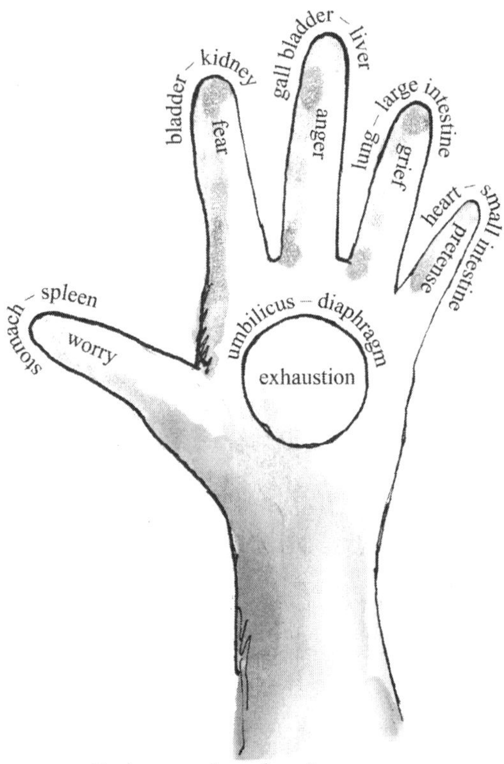

Each part of our hands governs organs that correspond to an attitude.

To a woman sitting next to me on a plane, trembling with fear, I took pleasure in whispering, "Hold your index finger." When I left my grief-stricken parents, it felt good to remind them, "Don't forget to hold your ring finger!" To a homeless man named Pascal whom I often ran into, it felt good to offer advice,

"You should hold your thumb for an hour every day."

It was all so simple. Too simple. How had I come up with all this? In some book of stories for children, like the ones I wrote?

So Jin Shin Jyutsu involved hands and breathing. Well, I knew all about breathing. I had done yoga, and I had been a smoker. I got into yoga to stop smoking. Most of all, I had suffered from terrible asthma. I knew what it was to be short of breath, to have tightness in the chest, and to go into apnea. I had known what breathing involved seemingly forever. Taking deep breaths and exhaling was sport for me.

I positioned my hands. I took a deep breath. My body gurgled in response. It gave me much joy. It was as simple as a haiku, that Japanese form of poetry that brings together nature and emotion in a single breath. The poet said, "Haiku *is*." Jiro Murai said, "Jin Shin Jyutsu *is*."

The tip of a blade of grass
Before the immensity of the sky
An ant

– *Hosai*[4]

Jin Shin Jyutsu helped me get past the first anniversary of my brother's death. My parents wept. They lay down and I placed my hands on their bodies, and we cried together. I had received no training, but I wasn't worried about hurting them. For Jiro Murai, Jin Shin Jyutsu is an effortless art. I performed it with the little knowledge I had of it and felt I could do no wrong. Since then, I have had hundreds of sessions and attended dozens of workshops, but I enjoy looking back on this time of innocence, for in it lay the journey that was about to unfold.

Of the Universe
An Explosion of the Ephemeral
Harmony

I started regular sessions with the practitioner-instructor, Natalie Max. Some days, I would fall asleep on her futon, other days I would take a nap in the movie theatre not far from her office. I learned that sleep, too, requires energy. I went there to recharge my batteries. With each successive appointment, I felt more relaxed, less anxious, and reassured. In November 2003, I attended my first five-day seminar. The instructor was an American, Wayne Hackett, whose background was in science and dentistry. He had learned Jin Shin Jyutsu from Mary Iino Burmeister. It was there I first saw pictures of Mary and her teacher, Jiro Murai, the two icons of the art, master and disciple, side by side. Mary, who was Japanese-American, had met the Master in Tokyo while with the post-war occupying forces under MacArthur. Murai Sensei asked, "Would you like to take a gift back to the West?" She studied under him until he died in 1960, following which she dedicated her life to developing Jin Shin Jyutsu and spreading knowledge of it throughout the United States and the world.

"It is not necessary to understand everything. One does better to take things one step at a time."[5] Mary knew well what she was talking about. At the end of the first workshop, I felt like a hiker at the foot of Mount Fuji. Much like the sacred mountain, Jin Shin Jyutsu towered over me, so beautiful, large, and mysterious that I felt irresistibly drawn to it. I did not know if I would ever make it to the top. I simply set out on the trail, alongside others, in all humility. That was fifteen years ago. Since then, I have ceased thinking about the mountaintop; I simply admire the mountain. I contemplate the scenery, caress the trunk of a thousand-year old tree, smell a flower, study the tracks of an animal, or add a rock to a cairn. And I write in my travel notebook and share my experiences with anyone who is interested.

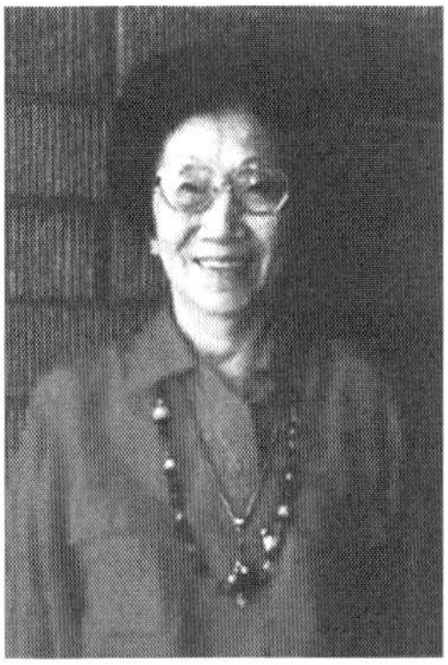

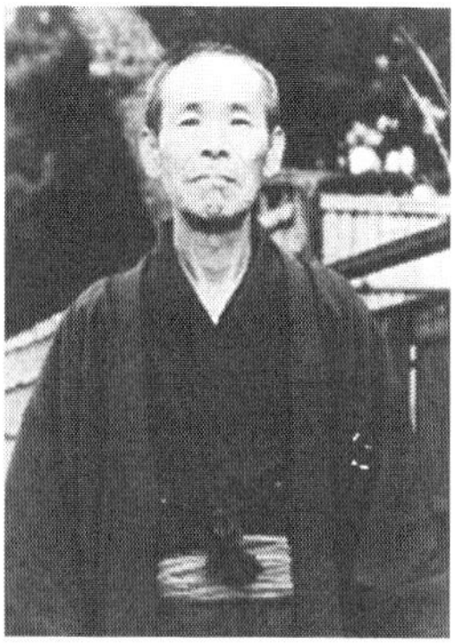

The teachings of Jin Shin Jyutsu are contained in two books, *Text 1* and *Text 2*, that students receive during their first five-day seminar. Leafing through the books one sees very few words. There are mostly drawings of the body, diagrams with dots that indicate where hands should be positioned to activate the flow of energy. There are twenty-six points called "safety energy locks" on either side of the body. Just as a torii deep in a thousand-year-old forest signals the presence of a shrine, each lock, designated by a number, is a gateway into the body. Each gateway tells the story of a particular pathway of energy. The pathways vary depending on which of the six depths they open onto, and whether the project for which we approach them is physical or emotional. Pulses tell us which pathway to choose. In Jin Shin Jyutsu workshops, the curriculum is always the same. The only variables are the instructor and the individual student's level of awareness. Students come from all walks of life. Men and women, both young and old, turn to Jin Shin Jyutsu after some trying experience or a long illness. Some are therapists, others come simply because they want to take care of their loved ones. Approaches can vary greatly depending on the instructors' nationality and training, and whether their background is in the sciences, philosophy, or the arts. Each of them has his or her own specific code: medicine, numerology, astrology, body movement, the study of sacred texts, the Bible, the Kabbalah, or Shinto mythology. In workshops, students are called upon both to give and to receive the art of Jin Shin Jyutsu several times a day.

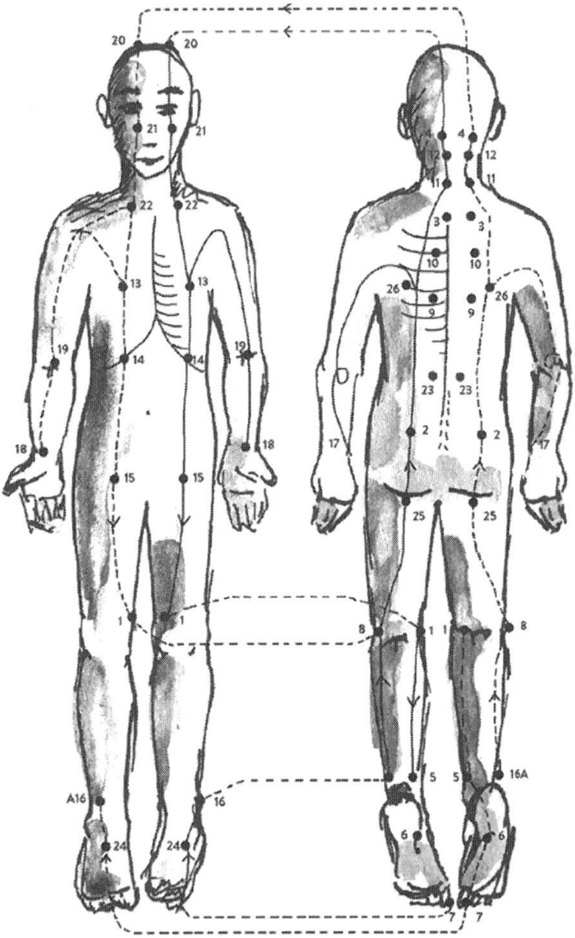

After drawings by Jiro Murai, as reprinted in a work by Haruki Kato[6]

From the most ancient traditions to modern-day physics, people have sought to understand what it is to be human. Their curiosity has led them to develop narratives. The art of Jin Shin Jyutsu is one of them. It tells of the journey of energy from the creation of the universe to the shaping of the Earth, of its transformation and densification. Mary Burmeister called it "the study of the depths." The depths are the qualities, the essences that constitute human beings. They are common to all of us whereas the emotional fabric of "who I am" is unique. The narrative that recounts the journey from formlessness to form can be viewed as "the soul's decision to become incarnated." As Matthias Roth said, "The process of incarnation continues well beyond birth ... At every point in our lives we make a new decision: How many I's will venture into the journey of life and thus into my body? The more we allow to go on this journey, the fuller our bodies and our lives."[7]

Starting at the very beginning, the ninth depth is considered the most distant, the original abyss in which neither space nor time existed, but which held the potential for all life, what Matthias Roth called "vastness." Then, suddenly, something happened: energy was concentrated into a dot. This is the eighth depth, the beginning of all things. The endlessly renewed energy of this eighth depth poured out with prodigious force, creating the sun in the seventh depth. Energy in the seventh depth is constant. It is the primordial life force, the light, the spark that gives life to our physical bodies. As we move from the sixth depth to the first, energy is gradually concentrated. This densified energy creates the harmony among the organs in the body, which evokes the marvelous connection between human beings and the universe.

In the seventh depth, the light from the sun enters the body at the level of the cervical spine, forming a six-pointed star. Saturn governs the first depth (Cervical 1). It is the primal cause: *Here I am. I am ME.* The stomach and the spleen are the organs associated with the first depth, which can be brought into harmony by holding the thumb. Venus governs the second depth (Cervical 5). It is the site of illuminating intelligence, wisdom, and love, which allow us to engage with another being: *There you are*. The lungs and the large intestine are the organs associated with the second depth, which can be brought into harmony by holding the ring finger. Jupiter governs the third depth (Cervical 2), the site of understanding, the swinging door that opens us to relationships. The liver and the gall bladder, which are associated with this depth, can be brought into balance by holding the middle finger. The fourth depth is governed by Mercury (Cervical 6) – *I have a destiny; I am growing; I am flourishing* – and is associated with the bladder and the kidney, which one brings into harmony by holding the index finger. Mars governs the fifth depth (Cervical 3) – *This is who I am. I can go wherever I want* – and is associated with the heart and the small intestine. The fifth depth is brought into harmony by holding the little finger. The moon governs the sixth depth (Cervical 7) – *I am perfectly balanced and in harmony. I am serene strength*. The umbilicus and the diaphragm are the organs of the sixth depth, which is brought into harmony by holding the palm of one's hand.

In this narrative, the body is a vessel into which energy flows. It is neither the primal source of energy nor a producer of energy. Jin Shin Jyutsu practitioners channel this universal energy by placing their hands on a patient's safety energy locks, much the way one uses jumper cables, as Mary Burmeister liked to say. The channeled energy revitalizes the body. Practitioners are not trying to do anything – which is not easy. They rather make it possible for something good to happen inside the patient by engaging a specific depth of the life force. Even when they are aware of a patient's symptoms, they do not treat the illness per se. Nor is it the goal of Jin Shin Jyutsu to replace medical assistance or medicine. Practitioners rather consider the person as a whole and seek to identify points of the body through which to promote self-regulation. They harmonize the physical and emotional functions so as to allow energy to follow its natural path.

This art of happiness, also called the art of longevity or the art of benevolence, was passed down from generation to generation over many centuries in Japan before falling into oblivion. The energy narrative can still be found in Shinto worship practiced today, personified in myth. I, along with hundreds of other pilgrims, bowed before the temple at Ise Jingu dedicated to the goddess Amaterasu, the Sun, the imperial family's ancestor. In Shingu, I climbed the five hundred thirty-eight steps of Mount Gongen to place my hand on the rock of the gods, where Izanami and Izanagi, Amaterasu's parents, first set foot on the Earth. On the pilgrimage routes in Kumano, I drank water from the sacred waterfall on Nachi-san, the tallest uninterrupted waterfall of the archipelago, the source of all sources.

In Jin Shin Jyutsu, we speak not of illnesses but of projects. An illness is a label. Thousands of people may have been given the same label but the state of their energy is in no two cases alike. Projects are the result of the disharmonious way energy is circulating in the body. "We need never know fatigue," Mary said. "Energy can never be tired. It is our personal imbalance that causes fatigue."[8] Beyond every disharmony lies the memory of the universal energy, the energy of life beyond form. When the body is in chaos because the flow of energy has stagnated, or reversed course, or divided into several pathways, reactivating the energy flow can restore order and harmony.

Jin Shin Jyutsu has become part of who I am. It is now an art of living, a second language for me. It has taught me to know myself, helped me rid myself of my fears, and made the invisible visible. Thanks to this art of compassion, I am now able to be genuinely present, to be truly there for a person in pain. When a passerby fainted in the street, I held his ring finger until the paramedics arrived. When a close family member was in a coma, I held his big toes and talked to him for an hour. I held the calves of a friend who was undergoing chemotherapy and showed an inconsolable child how to hug and comfort herself. When I found myself confronted by someone in a rage, rather than argue, I held his middle finger in my mind.

Jin Shin Jyutsu tells us that life is a journey that allows us to experience consciously a state of being. By setting a single intention we can change our destiny.

When we travel, mere nothings – the look on someone's face, a few words floating in the air, a gesture of no consequence – become meaningful. Minute details can have an effect on travelers. Hold your index finger!

The Great Harmony!
The most secret of provinces
Hidden beneath the mountains,
Deep in the valley.
Oh, most charming of provinces!

– *Kojiki*[9]

II

The Key to Harmony

Japan
Unknown Planet
The Gateway

When I first arrived in Japan I was overwhelmed by a sensation unlike anything I had known, a feeling of happiness like no other.

It was an extraordinary experience. For hours, I found myself floating in a secret interval of time, in a void, in nothingness and impermanence. My suitcase was ridiculously large for the size of my bedroom, my lace-up shoes ridiculously inconvenient in a world where you constantly had to take them off. My mind was filled with practical information and cultural and intellectual knowledge that all proved utterly useless. I felt illiterate, disoriented, unsophisticated, and uncouth. I did not know the cultural codes and could not even fake knowing them. But for the first time in my life, having no grasp of a situation did not frighten me. I was able to let go.

Nowhere else in the world had I ever felt as light, as free to follow my intuitions, or as open to the poetry of life. My husband and I had been invited as writers; we could just go with the flow. Although nothing was familiar, we felt comfortable and derived pleasure from everything: the smell of a tatami, the steam from baths, the color of bento boxes, the obis on kimonos.

We spent the last three days of our trip in Kyoto. Our guide, Mr. Abe, wore a sheepskin jacket and never stopped laughing. He took us around the city in taxis driven by men wearing white gloves. Of all the temples we visited, all the bridges we crossed and the gardens we admired, the stone garden in Ryoan-Ji is the only place that made an indelible impression on me. It is a masterpiece of Zen culture, the guidebooks say, dating from the end of the 15th century. Fifteen stones, arranged from east to west in groups of five, two, three, two, and three, symbolize mountains floating on a layer of white gravel representing the ocean. I enjoyed counting the stones over and over, getting lost in their numbers, sketching them and their shadows, and retracing the lines the gardener-priest had raked into a ripple-like pattern. I was pleased to hear that Ryoan-Ji meant "Temple of the Peaceful Dragon" and pleased to reserve space in my imagination for this garden of meditation. We spent a very long time there trying to figure out how the rocks were laid out on the gravel. As our visit ended, Mr. Abe said, "Let's go to my house for tea."

Thus were we invited into someone's home, which is quite an honor. There was nothing unusual about the house. It was small and furnished as in the West. My attention was immediately drawn to an altar at the far end of the living room, a console table with an urn surrounded by several divinities, among which I recognized Buddha and the Virgin Mary. I stood gazing at the burning incense for so long that Mr. Abe eventually said, "That is my wife. She passed away on September 5th."

I felt a shudder run through me. That was the same day my brother died… Mr. Abe served tea and we chatted about this and that. He had been to France only once and stayed in a monastery near Montpellier. I asked him: "Do you mean you learned your excellent French from monks who had taken a vow of silence?" He laughed, then went to get first one, then a second lacquered box from a cabinet.

"I have gifts for you," he said.

Each box held hundreds of slips of paper. Those in the box on the right had writing in kanji, those on the left, Roman script. Mr. Abe asked us our birthdays, then handed us each two pieces of paper, with December 1 for Daniel and April 27 for me. The one I could read began with *"Hail Mary full of grace."* I noticed that the spelling of the word "womb" had been corrected and was quite moved by that. "What is on the other one?" I asked. "A Buddhist prayer," Mr. Abe answered.

My senses awakened. "Do you write down these prayers every day?" Mr. Abe told us that every morning he woke up at four, went to his desk, and copied the Buddhist prayer and then the *Hail Mary*. He then read them aloud in a single breath, after which he would drink his first cup of tea of the day. I was exultant. I was about to gain access to the spiritual world I had been yearning for ever since Thierry died.

I asked one question after another: "How long have you been doing this? Does this date to your time in the monastery? Or to Mrs. Abe's illness? Why do you do it? Why the *Hail Mary* and the Buddhist prayer? How many boxes do you have? Is this Japanese tradition?"

Mr. Abe was unperturbed. He remained silent for a moment, then looked directly at us and said: "I started this ritual four years ago."

Four years ago. Why then? What happened?

Seated in the little house in Kyoto, near the altar with the urn holding his wife's ashes amid the various divinities, Mr. Abe remained silent while I peppered him with questions. We waited impatiently, I, for the moment when he would make *the* revelation that would serve as a beacon in my spiritual quest. He took a few sips of tea, then turned to me, having at last decided to speak. Carefully pronouncing each word, he said: "I have been doing this since I stopped smoking!" It was hardly the answer I had hoped for. But what kind of reply had I been expecting? Mr. Abe had stopped smoking. I had, too, and I remembered well how difficult that was. He had taken to writing prayers and reading them aloud. Why not? Suddenly his answer shot through me like a fault through the Earth's crust. He was Japanese. This was a lesson for the Westerner I am who believes that every question has an answer.

Back in France, I enjoyed telling this story to friends, emphasizing all the things that distinguish Eastern thinking from the way we think in the West. Months went by. The following summer, a friend of Mr. Abe's came to visit. He had heard of our trip to Kyoto. We learned from him that Mr. Abe had invited us into his home because we had astounded him. He had never, ever, met anyone like us. We were foreigners, tourists, and he had taken us to exceptional sites, yet never once did we take a photograph. We were an enigma to him. It was not a conscious decision, but I had stopped taking pictures after my brother died. Daniel didn't take pictures, either.

During dinner that evening, we once again told the story of what happened in Mr. Abe's house and I apologized to his friend. How could I have been so inconsiderate as to ask all those questions? I had been such a boor!

Then I got to the end of the story: "… since I stopped smoking."

Everyone burst out laughing.

Only Mr. Abe's friend did not react.

He had undoubtedly found it terribly insensitive of me to tell perfect strangers an intimate story that centered on Mrs. Abe's death. I had followed one gaffe with another. I was really embarrassed.

A little later, as our guest was about to leave, he whispered to me, "There is something I have to tell you." He looked solemn, ill at ease, almost tormented. "I have known Mr. Abe for more than thirty years," he said. "Abe-san never smoked."

After this incident, I found myself captivated by Japan. Mr. Abe had placed a towering torii in my personal landscape, like the torii in Oyunohara.

Ten years went by. I was studying Jin Shin Jyutsu and at the same time becoming increasingly passionate about Japanese culture and history. I made Japanese friends and started thinking about going back, this time with a writing project.

People who speak of Japan frequently evoke the importance there of form and esthetics. I wanted to find out what lay behind them, how that same sensitivity manifests itself in the way they take care of their bodies, and how it affects the mind and the spirit. I decided to do research on Jiro Murai, to whom we owe this thousands-of-years-old art of healing called Jin Shin Jyutsu, this "physio-philosophy" that teaches us to know ourselves.

In 2017, everything was in place for me to carry out my plan. The journey began in March, when I landed in Tokyo. I thought I had learned how to pronounce "Jin Shin Jyutsu" correctly, yet none of the Japanese I spoke with had ever heard of it. No one knew what I was talking about. No one recognized the name Jiro Murai, who didn't even have a Wikipedia article. I was flabbergasted.

Who was Jiro Murai? He was the man who said, "Everything is contained in the breath. Through a process of densification and dissolution, the breath is the ultimate healer." As if that helped! Where was I to start? All at once the Abe conundrum came back to me. "I have been doing this since I stopped smoking!" he said. "Abe-san never smoked," countered his friend. Every morning, Abe-san wrote down his prayers, a Buddhist prayer in Japanese, *Hail Mary* in French, then read them aloud, in one breath. I don't read Japanese, but I remembered the *Hail Mary*. I recited it, in one breath, the way Mr. Abe had, then repeated it ten times. The hidden meaning of the words suddenly became clear. I breathe in and receive, I breathe out and the prayer helps diffuse the breath so deep down within me that it regains strength and travels back up. "Since I stopped smoking" simply referred to breathing, to the magic of breath. The breath that lies at the origin of life and that generates movement; the breath that travels down the front of the body, all the way to the big toes, and moves back up the back, bringing together heaven and Earth. It cleans away "dust, dirt, and greasy grime," as Mary Burmeister so often put it. The more deeply we breathe the lighter we become. Breathing solidifies and dissolves, generates and regenerates. It allows us to connect with the energy of the universe.

That day, for the first time, I became aware of those few seconds between exhaling and inhaling during which the void is, when nothingness is, when there is neither thought nor evidence of anything, that space where human beings are ONE with the universe. I was reminded of a verse in the Bible – Matthew 16:19 – that Mary Burmeister often cited: "I will give you the keys of the kingdom of heaven, and whatever you shall bind on earth shall have been bound in heaven, and whatever you shall loose on earth shall have been loosed in heaven."[10] Aha! Breathing was the key.

Whether we are aware of it or not, in those few seconds between exhaling and inhaling we are suspended in an eternity in which anything is possible, in which any transformation can occur, in which the visible becomes invisible, in which negative thoughts become positive, and illness becomes healing.

The intimacy with which the body is cared for runs as deep as the intimacy with faith. My journey could begin.

"For many centuries the key to the treasures of Jin Shin Jyutsu was passed from generation to generation by verbal teachings. Gradually these keys began to fade until the true concept of this art was virtually lost." Mary Burmeister wrote: "The rediscovery of these ancient treasures came about by Master Jiro Murai of Japan, in the early 1900's."[11]

My friend Kyoko Watanabe joined me on the search for Master

Jiro Murai. We had only a few clues to start with: a name, two dates, three locations, not exactly what you would need to write a novel. I would simply have to explore the shadow he cast beneath the square light of the moon.

To be one with one's breath is never to go against what comes your way, but rather always to go along with it.

In my hermitage
The square light of the moon
At my window

– *Basho*[12]

In your eyes
I sense a mystery
What mystery is hidden therein?

– *Kojiki*[13]

III

Following Jiro Murai's Shadow One Step at a Time

Kaga
Mountains and Sea
The Source

The advice given to anyone struggling with writer's block, my friend and guide tells me as the northbound *shinkansen* speeds out of Tokyo, is to go to an *onsen*. In Japanese, there are a number of ways to say 'I', depending on whether the person speaking is young or old, wealthy or poor, male or female. In 1905, Natsume Soseki's *I Am a Cat* caused quite a humorous stir when he endowed the cat with the "I" of a nobleman. The "I" here, my "I," is that of a French woman, a writer, who has been practicing self-help Jin Shin Jyutsu for fifteen years and has set out in search of Japan by following the path taken by Jiro Murai, a man of wisdom, a healer, and a doctor, whose official biography is but a few lines long.

I am heading for the town of Kaga Onsen, in Ishikawa Prefecture. According to his disciple, Haruki Kato, this is where Jiro Murai was born in 1886, during the Meiji era. Located on the west coast of Japan, facing toward China, not far from Kanazawa, Kaga and its famous hot springs are a veritable paradise for thermal bath lovers. The old section of town owes its name to the Daishoji River. The houses there were all built with a view of Hakusan, the White Mountain with its eternal snows. Today, Hakusan is hidden by clouds as the train pulls in through paddy fields whose green shoots of rice have barely begun pushing up through the damp soil. Ah, the smell of rice! It is absolutely everywhere, seeping out from the bentos at lunchtime. I first smelled it when I landed in Narita. It was perceptible even in the airport's aseptic air. It was my first sensory experience, and the subject of my first conversation as well, which I had with Misako Nemoto, a friend of Kyoko Watanabe's and she, too, a professor at Meiji University in Tokyo. From her wonderful article on glutinous rice I remember this: "We need to moisten our thoughts more, as we do our food, which is why most Asians eat rice." Kyoko still recalls how surprised she was when she first came across an ad in France touting non-sticky rice. Then she mentions *onigiri,* those little handmade rice balls formed by pressing the palms together in a gesture, *nigiru,* known for its energy-giving virtues. I smile. This is exactly the kind of information I was hoping to gather. In Jin Shin Jyutsu, bringing your hands together is a way of stimulating the main central flow of energy that rises along the spine, travels over the head, moves down through the sternum to the pubic bone, and then rises again at the back, making an oval circuit. As I thank my friend for this insight, I realize that when the Japanese bow with their hands pressed together and their knees close to each other, as is the custom, they are unknowingly seeking a connection to the cosmic source. *Arigato! Arigato gozaïmas! Thank you. Thank you very much. Thank you so much.* These are the first words I have managed to pick out from the muddle of chatter I hear. I enjoy repeating them as I try to pronounce them correctly and respectfully and remain fully present, whether I am thanking someone for a great favor or a small kindness. It is not at all a half-hearted "thank you" that is conventional or simply polite, or affected, or bombastic. It is a "thank you" I pronounce as I bow and breathe out, like a sacred mantra passing over my lips.

It is mid-March and the forecast calls for snow or, at best, rain. The midday sky is low and grey when a golden 240-foot statue with a baby in her arms appears, looming over the town like *Our Lady of the Guard,* in Marseille. It is Kannon Bosatsu, the Buddhist Goddess of Mercy. She stands facing the city of Osaka, home to the man who had it built. Had she stood guard over young Murai's dreams? Actually, she could not have. As I was later to learn, the statue was erected not that long ago, along with an amusement park. For now, it is enough for me to sense that I have come to a deeply inspiring place that brings together the two landscapes I treasure most: the ocean, like the one in my native Brittany, and the mountains, like those in the Vercors, my adopted home. In the Far East, mountains traditionally symbolize meditation, and the sea, compassion. Meditation is a matter of proper posture and finding one's center. Compassion is breathing in harmony with the ebb and flow of the waves. And in Japan, as everyone knows, where there is a mountain, the sea can't be far away.

As the bus bringing us from the station pulls in at the hotel, Kyoko points out a kimono shop across the street: Kato-Fashion Gallery. Kato, the owner's name, is the same as that of Haruki Kato, Jiro Murai's first disciple, and as that of Sadaki Kato, Haruki's son, who is an acupuncturist and Jin Shin Jyutsu practitioner. I had had a second appointment with him the day before, in his Tokyo office. I clearly needed two sessions of Jin Shin Jyutsu to get over my jetlag, empty my hard drive of all the political pollution that had filtered into it during the election campaigns in France, and to open my synapses fully so that I could understand this world so radically different from the West. Sadaki Kato knelt on the tatami while I lay on a futon. He listened to my pulses on the right and left wrists, the superficial and the deep pulses. I did not ask him what he heard, nor which flow he was going to do to reduce my fatigue and clear my lungs. He placed his hands on my fully dressed body without applying pressure or massaging. After about an hour-long session, he listened to my pulses again.

I was to never be the same. I would no longer stumble over slippers, or come out of the bathroom in bathroom slippers, or out of the toilet in toilet slippers. I would never forget to remove my indoor slippers before stepping onto the bedroom tatami in my socks. I would become expert with chopsticks in getting a piece of tofu out of a broth, and would no longer yank the sliding doors open. I would keep to the left in the subway corridors and the escalators in Shibuya and Shinjuku. I would no longer have my head in the clouds, and Kyoko would no longer impishly chide me, "But I already told you..."

The young and pretty Saki, one of my friend Michèle Mizubayashi's students, accompanied me to my first appointment with Sadaki Kato. Her mission was to guide the illiterate I was through the forest of *kanji, hiragana* and *katakana* (– the three Japanese writing systems consisting of Chinese characters, *kanji,* and two alphabets of phonetic syllables, *hiragana* and *katakana* ... all of which makes the language delightfully complex). We did not have an address – the GPS has got to be a Japanese invention – but Mr. Kato had sent a map of the neighborhood and a picture of his apartment house. I don't know more than a few words in Japanese, among them "Jin Shin Jyutsu," and not a single person I met had ever heard of it. Sadaki Kato explained that his father, Haruki, who was Murai's only heir in Japan, had been too ill to teach. He was able to pass on his art only to his wife, who died prematurely, and himself, his son.

Kato-Sensei did, though, publish a book that is still in print. Kyoko picked up a copy before I arrived. It has Murai's teachings but just about no biographical material. I might as well be looking for a needle in a haystack! Except that right then I am in Japan, strolling with Saki through Rikugien Garden, going on and on about the French filmmaker Eric Rohmer. I notice a gardener plucking at a tuft of pine needles and another one filing down bark on a branch. There are so many ways to tend to your garden! I am deeply touched by what I see. The trees are so well treated. They are swathed, guided, surrounded by elaborate structures to protect against heavy snowfalls, held upright with stakes, coddled, and cared for. Gardening in empathy with nature.

On my second appointment, Sadaki invites Kyoko to sit in on the session. They speak Japanese with each other. When we leave, Kyoko is reassured. Mr. Kato is neither a poser nor a charlatan. He is a therapist with several strings to his bow, two of which, acupuncture and moxibustion – a technique that involves stimulating acupuncture points by heating them with moxa, small cones of burning dried, ground Artemisia, or mugwort – are widely known.

Divine Tree
Temple Gate
Salutation

Planting a single cypress is like planting a hundred trees, said a bonze in an inspired talk given in honor of the goddess Amaterasu in 717. On the heights of Yamanaka Onsen, four cypress trees stand guard over a small Shinto temple. The site is called Kayano Osugi, *osugi* meaning, aptly, "tall cypress," and *kayano* "one hundred." I immediately leaned my back against one of them and inhaled deeply to breathe in the magic power samurai warriors drew in. Before I left France, Rose, six years old, had made me watch her favorite animated film, *Totoro*. And there we were, Kyoko and I, wide-eyed with wonder, just like Satsuki and Mei, the two little girls in the film who stand in awe at the foot of a giant tree in front of their new house. To capture the moment, I took a picture of Kyoko, her slender frame seemingly disappearing into the mass of the two-thousand-year-old trunk. Before leaving Tokyo, we had strolled through the charming, narrow streets of Ogiku-bo. A shopkeeper having sung the praises of cypress wood, I bought a small cutting board with lace-like natural grain. Cypress wood is valued as a protection against mold. As we were about to leave the apartment, we set a lemon and a clementine on the board. When we returned, the fruit was unspoiled.

I love trees, and have ever since I was a child roaming through the countryside with my grandmother. She taught me how to recognize the bark of different trees and the shape of their leaves. She wasn't going to let her granddaughter mistake a chestnut tree with the delicious chestnuts we used to roast in the fireplace for a horse chestnut tree, like the one in the schoolyard, with conkers you put in drawers to ward off moths. I have loved trees ever since I watched my father plant woods around the family home in Brittany, ever since I decided to plant some trees myself, watched them grow in the arid soil of the Vercors: the beeches, maples, ashes, pines, hazelnuts, lilacs, and elderberries that we got from a nearby forest when they were just saplings; the birches that were already fairly tall when we bought them, and the giant among them, my goddaughter Anna's linden tree. Every August, the three of us, Anna, I, and the linden tree, pose for a picture. And with every passing year we can see the foliage thicken, the young girl becoming a young woman, and me, as I…

I bow to those trees every time I go back. They are over twenty years old now, and I thank them for having withstood the wind and the snow.

神木
The Divine Tree

The Kayano Osugi cypress trees
are over two thousand years old!

A family of giants rises 180 feet into the air. A *shimenawa,* a rope of braided rice straw, has been tied around each of them to mark it as sacred. The cypress is the tree of life and the symbol of immortality, and every civilization recognizes its spiritual qualities. In the Shinto "religion," *hinoki* is used for temples, priests' staffs, and ritual fire. But what is Shintoism? In the ten years I had known Kyoko we had never talked about religion. When I was staying with her, I would watch her, every morning, pause a moment before the little altar dedicated to her beloved mother, the writer Yoko Mochizuki. She would burn incense and make an offering: a book, a flower, a small bowl of rice, a kaki, or simply a glass of water. We were on the road, but I was sure that every morning she paused before that little altar in her mind. Is ancestor worship Shinto or Buddhist? That was when I understood that to be Shinto is to be Japanese, and to be Japanese is to be Shinto.

The Kayano Osugi cypress trees were planted a thousand years before the *Kojiki* was written ("Records of Ancient Matters," a collection of myths and legends on the origin of the Japanese archipelago, composed in 712), a time when the Japanese worshipped *kami*: energies, spirits, and forces superior to human beings. There were said to be as many as eight million of them, the number 8 symbolizing a multitude in Japanese mythology. Kami were incarnations of mountains, tigers, snakes, even the emperor himself. They were said to reside in the heavens, but they often came down to Earth to visit shrines. The Kayano Osugi cypress trees, with their *shimenawa* tied around them, are *yorishiro*, which means they are able to attract kami and shelter them. Kami are neither intrinsically good nor bad, but they are capable of getting angry, and inspire a feeling of respectful awe. People pray to them to have their wishes granted. They make offerings to them and clap their hands twice to draw their attention.

Having been imported from China and Korea between the 5th and 6th centuries, the Kayano Osugi cypress trees saw the arrival of Buddhism in Japan. Here, on the shores of the Sea of Japan, the eight-hundred-year-old trees watched over the benevolent welcome given to this path to wisdom that has so profoundly enriched life and art on the archipelago.

With the arrival of Buddhism came Japan's discovery of the kanji, which the Japanese adapted to develop a writing system of their own. The *Kojiki* is in fact the first book written in Japanese. Before 712, writers expressed themselves exclusively in Chinese. Along with Buddhism came calligraphy, painting, architecture, tea, Chinese medicine, and the mudras. Buddhism first appeared in the 6th century before our era in India, where it was declared a state religion in 592. From the outset, and up until the Meiji era (mid-nineteenth century), Buddha and the kami got along so well that they inhabited the same temples.

The Kayano Osugi cypress trees were 1,800 years old when the Spanish missionary Saint Francis-Xavier came from Lisbon to Kagoshima in 1549 and brought Christianity to Japan. This was the time of the Portuguese Society of Jesus and the Spanish Mendicant Orders, and the time known as the Nanban Trade Period as well. All of which was to last barely a century. In 1650 the isolationist laws known as *Sakoku* were implemented. Nearly all Europeans were expelled, and Christians were martyred for their beliefs. These events are depicted in *Silence*, a historical novel written by a Catholic author, Shusaku Endo, and adapted for the screen by Martin Scorcese in 2016. In the Kutani Porcelain Art Museum in Daishoji, our guide showed us a porcelain dish from that era. For the Christians hiding in the region the vine stock painted on it represented the Cross. They would pray to it in secret.

The Kayano Osugi cypress trees were almost two thousand years old when, in 1689, they were visited by Matsuo Kinasaku, known as Basho. This master of the haiku was an itinerant poet. He spent nine days in Yamanaka Onse. It was here that he separated from his companion and disciple, Sora, who was said to be ill. And it was here, too, that Basho learned of his own approaching death, which was to occur five years later, in 1694, in Osaka. And it was also here, legend says, that his fascination with the beauty of a seventeen-year-old boy inspired him to write the following verse (it was thought that a chrysanthemum decoction could restore youth):

Waters of Yamanaka
Fountain of youth, here
No need for chrysanthemums

–*Basho*[14]

The Kayano Osugi cypress trees were immortalized in 1930 when they were designated a natural treasure. In 1945, homage was paid to them by Emperor Showa (1901-1989), the one hundred and twenty-fourth Emperor of Japan and the last of the divine-right emperors. When he traveled through the region two years later, this descendent of the sun goddess, Amaterasu, had already had to deal with the tragic earthquake that devastated Tokyo in 1923, the war in Manchuria, the attack on Pearl Harbor, and the bombing of Hiroshima and Nagasaki. His reign was to be the longest in the history of the Land of the Rising Sun.

神殿
Temple

With Kyoko Watanabe by my side, I walked up the alley lined with cypress trees to a little shrine edged with snow and guarded by two sculptures of dogs, *komainu*. I purified myself at the *chozusha*, or 'small fountain'. I poured a small ladleful of water over my hands, first the left, then the right, then poured a little more into the palm of my left hand and raised it to my lips.

I bowed before the torii.

At the entrance to the temple, I put down a small coin as an offering. It was a 50-yen piece with a hole in the middle you could see through, like a symbol of the connection with the universe. I rang the bell to alert the gods to my presence.

I bowed twice, fully mindful as I did, and breathed in, breathed out, breathed in, breathed out.

I clapped my hands twice. A hundred temples later, at Ise Jingu, I would see pilgrims spread their arms to open their chests wide and clap their hands loudly, and I would do the same.

I bowed once more.

As I stood beneath the Kayano Osugi cypress trees I could feel the essence of Japan permeate my being. I could not help but think that as Jiro Murai worked to bring the art of longevity he named Jin Shin Jyutsu back to the world he must have been carrying the tree of life, the Kayano Osugi *hinoki,* in the depths of his heart.

Posthumous Name
From One Shore to Another
DNA of the Soul

The fog had begun to blanket the tops of the cypress trees. At the bus stop at the foot of Kayano Osugi, Kyoko was keeping watch. On the way out, the driver had made a point of telling us the exact time of the last stop of the day. We got there early. The temperature had dropped and we were anxious to get back to the hotel.

There was not a soul in sight.

The evening before we left, as we watched a game show on television, *Are you Cat or Dog*? I realized that the majority of Japanese people identify with cats. Yes indeed, the Japanese are very much cat-like. When they fall asleep on trains, meticulously wash up at baths, even when they ride their bikes there is a feline quality to what they do. In Yasujiro Ozu's films, which I can watch over and over, I love to watch them walk, bow, stand motionless, get down on their knees, lie down on a tatami and get back up, slide doors open or closed, hold little bowls in the palm of their hands as they drink, delicately pick up pieces of food with chopsticks… every one of these gestures as perfectly choreographed as a dance.

"You are obviously free to do whatever you want, said the cat, Otsuka, as it carefully licked one of its paws, but I think you should show a little more consideration for your shadow. It might actually be ashamed to be diminished like that. I know if I were your shadow I would not appreciate being reduced to half my size."[15]

Like many Japanese writers, Haruki Murakami has no qualms about having cats speak. Now that Perlette, a stray cat I picked up in the country, is a part of my life, I understand that this intimate connection with animals is not just the stuff of fiction. The company of cats teaches us a lot about the shadow of things, and about all the things we cannot see. In Hiraide Takashi's novel, *The Guest Cat*,[16] the mysterious and beautiful Chibi is portrayed as the incarnation of the garden's soul.

Still no bus.

We were in the part of Japan where Basho and his companion Sora, who had been traveling on foot together, went their separate ways. Ever since I learned that *basho* means "banana plant" I have felt closer to the poet, and to haiku as well. After Basho retreated to a hermitage one of his disciples gave him a banana plant. The so-called "tallest herb in the world" dies after producing its fruit, then comes back to life. When Basho, then a monk, took this name he must have known that the Buddha had made the banana plant the symbol of instability, vulnerability, and the vanity of material things.

"What is a haiku, exactly?" Terada Torahiko asked his professor, Natsume Soseki. "It is a universe that radiates outward from a focal point, much like the pivot pin that holds the slats of a hand fan together," was the reply.[17] When I read this, I immediately thought of the safety energy locks in Jin Shin Jyutsu, which Jiro Murai called "energy points" (*kiten*). Like any well-educated person in Japan, he had surely practiced the art of the haiku. Jin Shin Jyutsu is, the haiku *is*, life *is*. The practice of Jin Shin Jyutsu is similar to that of the haiku in that it allows us all to be artists, to experience the interpenetration of the eternal and the ephemeral that nature brings out in us, and allows us to express what we see or feel through what Roland Barthes called a "thin horizon of words."[18]

Born into a family of samurai, in 1644, near *Iga Ueno,* Basho was contemporary to the French playwright Jean Racine and the poet Jean de la Fontaine. He dedicated his life to teaching and travel. After taking the monk's robe, he set off on a journey across Japan. It was here, 1,400 miles later, after his companion, Sora, had left him, that he came to know solitude.

俳句
Haiku

But unlike Basho I found myself filled with joy, peace, and confidence here. Kyoko was with me. She and I had met in 2006 when my husband, who like me is a writer, was invited to Japan and I came along. Kyoko was his interpreter and took the time to show us around. As we strolled through the Jinbo-cho quarter and looked in shop windows, I was amazed to find a Japanese version of *J'aime* (*I Love*),[19] a children's book I had written and which Natali Fortier had illustrated. Kyoko was thrilled for me. I gave her a copy of the book, and she has treasured it ever since.

I had been doing Jin Shin Jyutsu for only three years but I took that moment as a sign that I would come back to this country. Kyoko Watanabe was to become a part of our lives, just as Michèle and Akira Mizubayashi were to. For the past few years, she has stayed with us every September when she comes to Paris. When she first visited France, with her parents, she was just twelve years old. At the beginning of our travels together, I knew little of her beyond her deep knowledge of French culture and her wonderful gift for connecting with people of all kinds. When I first spoke to her of my project, she had never heard of Jin Shin Jyutsu or of Jiro Murai, either. Nor had she ever set foot in this part of Japan, but she was game.

"When you travel, you need a companion, but in life, what you need is compassion," Sakura said to Kafka Tamura, quoting a Japanese proverb.[20] In Kyoko I had found a companion who empathized with my ignorance. She could see what I was seeing for the first time, hear what I needed to understand, and translate what I barely managed to articulate. She was engaged in my quest, at my side with every step I took and with every emotion I felt. "Even chance encounters stem from happenings in our previous lives," one reads in one of Haruki Murakami's works.[21] I like to think that Kyoko is my little Japanese sister and that we are connected through the DNA of our souls.

The bus never came.

We had to call the hotel to get a taxi. On an impulse, as we were driving alongside a cemetery, I asked Kyoko to stop. It was a small, country cemetery on a hillside. It was the second one I had visited, the first being the one in Tokyo, in the Sugamo district, where Mr. Kato's clinic is located. After the second session, Kyoko wanted to show me a statue of the Buddhist deity Jizo, the Protector of Children. Contrary to all the other Jizos I was to see subsequently – all of them tiny stone sculptures – this one was a huge bronze statue with a red bib. I stopped to put down an offering. There was a boy of nine or ten next to me, bent over at the waist. He was bowing to the Protector of Children! When he picked up his backpack to leave, we followed him through a maze of tiny streets out to a cemetery. From afar, I watched him burn a few sticks of incense at a family gravesite. Had he lost his father or his mother? His grand-parents? A brother or a sister? Graves are graves, and the ones here are not unlike ours, not unlike the one where my brother and father are buried in the small town of Plogonnec, near Quimper. The lone difference is the presence of long wooden slats (*sotoba*) leaning against the tombstones. In Japan, people have only one first name, which changes after death, and it is their posthumous name that is carved on the wooden boards.

Kyoko was suddenly very exited. She wanted to show me the kanji on a gravestone. "Look, it says Murai!" I took a picture of the characters set off against a black background. This was a Murai family gravesite. Chiseled into the granite above the ideogram were three triangles in a circle, a family crest, perhaps. The emblem of the imperial family is a sixteen-petal chrysanthemum.

Three triangles...

I was to find the same geometrical pattern on Enoshima Island, across from Tsujido, where Jiro Murai is said to have spent the last part of his life. There, it represented the *mon*, or crest, of the Hojo clan, an important samurai family who dominated Japan during the Kamakura Period (12th to 14th centuries) when a variety of schools of Buddhism were established, Zen being one of them.

The Murai gravesite featured a lotus blossom above the circle with the three triangles. The lotus is an aquatic plant that emerges from muddy murkiness to yield a flower of divine beauty. It represents the evolution of the soul and the possibility for every human being to attain Buddhahood after death, whatever the person's life has been. On the stone above the lotus was a mantra invoking trust in Buddha, *Namu Amida Butsu*, which leads me to believe that the three triangles in the circle were probably a Buddhist *yantra*. Just as a mantra is a vocal support for meditation, a *yantra* is a visual one, and both serve to help us meditate as we seek to open ourselves to the forces of the cosmos. The circle is the *chakra*, the element of air; a triangle pointing downward is *Shakti kona*, feminine energy, water; and a triangle pointing upward is Shiva kona, masculine energy, fire. *Yantras* are gateways or pathways that lead from the manifest (*Shakti*) to the non-manifest (*Shiva*). They weave a fabric of consciousness, forming a kind of energy web. To meditate is to be with one's breath. Jin Shin Jyutsu tells us that to be with the breath is to bring heaven down to Earth. Through processes that densify and dissolve, the breath is the ultimate healer.

All these symbols are like keys that help us navigate through time and across civilizations, from the most ancient animist or Celtic traditions to Judaism and Christianity, from Pythagoras to Plato and Leonardo da Vinci, and so on.

The circle and the sphere represent the infinite, perfection, the divine. Plato called them perfect shapes. Everything that is animate, especially if in a spherical form, appertains to the soul. Planets rotate in regular orbits that obey the laws of circles and spheres. And this Law of Harmony applies to the human soul as well.

The triangle represents the Holy Trinity, unity.

The square represents the material world, life on Earth.

There are no chance encounters.

That gravesite, even if not that of Jiro Murai's family, was a marker on the path leading to him. The year of his death is known, but the exact date and site where he is buried are not. He lived to be seventy-four. Two years prior to his death, which he had foreseen by carefully listening to his pulses, he named his disciple, Haruki Kato, the Japanese heir to Jin Shin Jyutsu. Jiro Murai is known as a practitioner of oriental medicine. During the eight years Haruki Kato spent with him, his mentor rarely spoke about his life and was extremely discreet about all things personal. He did not leave enough for a biography, and certainly not enough for there to develop any kind of personality cult.

Life is a journey that allows us to experience a state of being, Jiro Murai's teachings tell us. As I was writing these lines, I received an email from Kyoko reminding me that it was May 16th, known in Japan as Travel Day, "because it is the day the great poet Basho set off on his long trek."

First Bath
Main Central Vertical
Kimono

We had to go through two doors to get into our room, first a sliding door, then, hidden behind it, a swing door with a lock, the kind you find in hotels everywhere. As we entered we were struck by the pungent smell of green rice straw, the smell of tatamis. A narrow entryway with a wood floor led to the bathroom and the toilet. This was where you were supposed to take your shoes off before stepping onto the tatami. There were six of them in the bright, virtually barren room with a lone lacquered table with cushions around it in the middle. I saw nothing resembling a bed that we could stretch out on, which would have been welcome after the full day we had had. At the far end, a papered sliding panel obscured the window, and in front of us, in an area one step down, were a table and two chairs. I was very tempted to sit down in the *tokonoma* – but that isn't done – , an alcove a little higher than the tatamis, decorated with a hanging scroll and a vase but with neither bench nor shelves. In *In Praise of Shadows*, Junichiro Tanizaki (1886-1965) describes it as "a recessed space where filtered rays of light create patches of darkness."[22]

It was time to put away my luggage and clothes. Behind sliding doors lined with thick paper with a plum tree motif there was a closet meant for just that. In the baskets on the shelves were Japanese clogs and a number of *yukata*, cotton kimonos of various colors. Every person I saw in this bath-hotel was wearing one. It is traditional Japanese attire worn by men and women alike, and literally means, "the things we wear."

Since we could not flop down on a mattress, Kyoko and I decided to pay a visit to Mr. Kato's kimono shop across the street.

Ever since our first trip to Japan, Daniel has loved putting on a kimono in the morning when he writes. He owns several, but never seems to have enough of them. I had decided to bring him back a few more. One day, our friend Akemi who had been giving him kimonos for years asked, "Do you feel more centered when you have it on?"

Centered?

With its vertical lines, a kimono effectively induces us to stand straight, aligned with our axis.

着物
Kimono

Mr. Kato was not wearing a kimono in his shop; he was dressed in a suit. He wanted to know everything about me: where I came from, what I thought of Japan, if I was on vacation ... He was charming and funny. He was born here, but unfortunately had never heard of anyone named Murai. With regard to vacations, he told us that because he could not leave his store for stretches long enough to travel to distant lands he did his vacationing up on summits or down in the depths, mountain climbing or scuba-diving, always higher, always deeper.

I bought a *hanten* from him, a short quilted jacket like the ones people wear in the mountains in Japan. Mr. Kato would have liked to sell me as well clothes with blossom patterns or dragonflies, even a kimono that was outwardly plain but lined with rare silk, which is the height of elegance here, where people pay especial care to what others cannot see. Kimonos are T-shaped, with little regard for human anatomy. They are made of rectangular pieces of fabric, folded, sewn together, and held in place by a wide sash called an obi, which is tied at the back. The left panel is always laid over the right, except with the deceased, on whom it is the other way around. Mr. Kato thought us so nice that he gave us the address of his favorite restaurant, one that did not appear on the hotel's list, a place favored by locals and not frequented by tourists. He even drove us there in his car, a little box with four wheels like the ones you see in Japanese cartoons. We were greeted by Yuko, a handsome woman in her sixties dressed in a black kimono with a red obi. We took a seat at the bar alongside regulars who were watching a baseball game on TV. They struck up a conversation with us and gave us a glass of saké from their personal supply, a large flask they kept under the counter. We ended up having dinner at Yuko's every evening, and when the time came to say goodbye, we did so with a tinge of regret.

When we got back from the restaurant we found that the futons had been laid out on the tatami. Kyoko told me that it was possible to have five or six people sleeping in the same room. She was all excited. For her it was time to go to the baths. For me, it was my very first time to go to the baths. We put on our kimonos and our wooden clogs and headed down to the large hot water pool in the basement. Women of all ages were sitting around the steaming water on little wooden benches, soaping up, dousing themselves with water, scrubbing, shampooing, and rinsing themselves off. Only when they deemed themselves clean did they get into the pool and unwind, splashing around and giggling with their women friends. It was a moment of conviviality and pure happiness. Are there co-ed baths? Yes, there are. One of Kyoko's friends had been to one.

That night, I slept in my kimono. The futon floated about on the tatami like an unmoored raft. It was not up against a wall that I could lean on, as I am used to doing when I read or write in bed. With my body mellow from the bath, I felt I was drifting. The night I got to Tokyo, I was totally jetlagged, and when I tried to get up I literally had no sense of balance. There is a word for this in Japanese, but impossible to translate: *kanashibari*. *Kanashibari* often takes hold of you in the morning, when you are still half-asleep. You can't move your fingers, you feel you are glued to the futon, bolted to the tatami. Your ears start buzzing in a foreboding of the visions that follow: rounds of headless ghosts, creatures in the shape of black clouds penetrating deep within you, chickens sitting next to your face, deranged girls laughing… I tightened the obi on my kimono and focused on my daily Jin Shin Jyutsu practice, the Main Central Vertical. It is a self-help exercise that takes between thirty and forty minutes and revitalizes the entire body. Sometimes I fall asleep in the middle of it.

Self-Help
Main Central Vertical
Energy

1a.
I place the palm of my right hand on top of my head.

1b.
I place the fingers of my left hand between my eyebrows to regenerate the deep circulation of energy in the body and stimulate memory. This also allays senility.

2.
With my right hand still on my head, I place the fingers of my left hand on the tip of my nose to regenerate the circulation of the surface energy of the body as well as the reproductive functions.

3.
My right hand remains on my head. I place the fingers of my left hand on the sternum, between my breasts, to regenerate the energy of respiration (the lungs) and the pelvic girdle (the hips).

4.
My right hand still in place, I bring my left hand down to the base of the sternum, to the pit of the stomach. This regenerates the energy of the source of life, both its ascending and descending movements.

5.
I still have my right hand on my head. I lower my left hand and place it on the pubic bone to strengthen the spine.

6.
With my left hand on the pubic bone, I place my right hand at the base of the spine, on the coccyx, to regenerate the ascending energy and help circulation in the legs and feet.

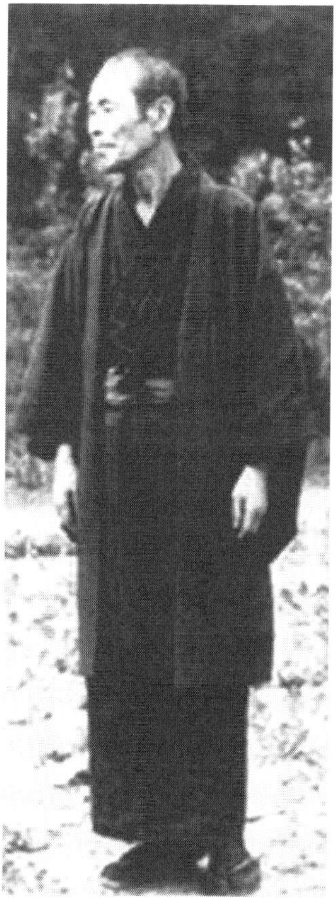

In the very few pictures we have of Jiro Murai he is always wearing a kimono. There is one full-length shot of him in a five-piece outfit, where he had put on a long jacket, a haori, over his kimono, which was of brown, or indigo, or perhaps black silk, and knotted with an obi.

He is in socks and sandals, and with his big toe separated from the others has a bit of a webbed-foot look. He is no longer a young man, but has the slim body and high forehead of a samurai. And his sober attire accentuates his elegance, natural authority, and nobility of soul. In another photo, an iconic close-up that Western instructors always place next to one of Mary Burmeister when they lead workshops, Murai Sensei is looking directly at the camera as if he had finally acceded to the photographer's request. He has his chin up in skeptical amusement and a somewhat impish look on his face (see page 23).

In yet another photograph, he is the only person wearing a kimono in a group of men and women dressed in Western clothes, among them Haruki Kato. It was probably taken at the end of a class, and dates from the late 1950s. Even though the kimono remains a traditional garment firmly rooted in Japanese culture, it ceased being everyday attire after the war. It is expensive and far too elaborate for modern life. Did Sensei Murai wear a kimono to distinguish himself from practitioners of Dutch medicine, which is what they call Western medicine here? Did he always dress that way or only on his monthly visits to Tokyo, when he came to practice his art and to teach? At that time, he was living in Tsujido, a seaside resort on the Pacific coast, on the bay of Sagami, across from the little island of Enoshima that one frequently sees in etchings. Today, Tsujido is just an hour's train ride from Shinjuku station in Tokyo. When Jiro Murai lived there, it was already a seaside resort catering to Tokyoites, but it was also home to a number of sanatoriums. Was Murai treating tuberculosis patients, tuberculosis being the great disease of the day? From the train window, you can see the ocean on one side and, when the skies clear after it rains, Mount Fuji on the other. I cannot imagine him driving a car in a kimono. For me, whatever is Japanese in the mystery of the art of Jin Shin Jyutsu is present in this garment.

Later, Kyoko would show me a picture of herself wearing the formal kimono handed down to her from her mother. The following year, at the graduation ceremonies at Meiji University, I admired the colors of the students' kimonos, each one more dazzling than the next.

Year of the Dog
Younger Brother
The Seventh Day

Jiro Murai was born into a family of doctors.

Traditional Japanese families had a predilection for naming their children according to their birth order: Taro or Ichiro for the oldest, Jiro for the second born, Kenshiro, the fourth one, Saburo for the youngest… to which could be added a prefix, as in Kojiro, Shinjiro, Yojiro, or even a zodiac sign like Usaburo (the third son, born in the year of the Rabbit). Lafcadio Hearn, a writer whose travels took him through Japan when Jiro Murai was still a child, observed the following: "For example, at meals, the oldest son is served first, followed by the second, the third, and so on, except when there is a really young child who can't wait. This custom has produced an amusing nickname for the youngest: Mr. Cold-Rice. Because he has to wait until his older brothers and the toddlers are served, when his bowl of rice finally reaches him it is usually ice cold."[23]

The name reveals the person, or so the saying goes. In all events, naming a newborn in Japan was a great responsibility entrusted to the father or grandfather, or in their absence, to the Shinto priest or a Buddhist monk. The family "name giving" ceremony, *Nazuke*, is usually held seven days after birth. Little Murai received the name Jiro, as did two of his contemporaries, Osaragi Jiro (1897-1973), the author of *47 Ronins*, and Yasujiro Ozu (1903-1963), the director of *Late Spring* and *Tokyo Story*, and Ichimongi Jiro, a character in Akira Kurosawa's masterpiece *Ran*, which was based on Shakespeare's *King Lear*.

The *Miyamairi*, or "shrine visit," takes place when the baby is around thirty days old. The mother, dressed in a formal kimono, carries the infant on her back swaddled in a newborn's kimono and held in place by a large swath of cloth. The entire household proceeds to the Shinto shrine to present the infant to the family's tutelary kami. The priest recites the ritual prayer and waves a sacred wand adorned with zigzagging paper streamers (*gohei*) above the infant's head to chase away whatever impurities might have come with him from the other world. Following the ceremony, the mother takes her baby from house to house, visiting friends and offering them candies (*ame*). In return, she receives small paper mache dogs, *Inu-Hariko*, that will watch over the child's health. The ceremonial day ends at the family home, where they are served a meal.

Like all Japanese babies, little Jiro was born with a blue spot on the lower part of his spine, on the sacrum. While I was working on this book, friends of Kyoko's, Kazumi and Yasuko, had a baby girl they named Madoka. I was quite touched when they asked me to come and look at the blue spot as they were about to change her diaper. "We know you are interested in everything Japanese. Would you like to see it?" It was a perfectly round, genuinely blue spot about the size of a thumbnail. It would disappear before the baby turned two. "*Madoka*, means round," Kazumi said, "like the moon or the universe."

As opposed to Western tradition, in Japan all birthdays are celebrated on the first day of the year. The minute a baby is born, he or she is already a year old. Those born on December 31st turn two the following day.

犬
Dog

"Mula-E-Jilo," as it is pronounced in Japanese, because the last name precedes the first and the 'r' is pronounced like an 'l', was born in 1886.

There is no mention anywhere of the month or the day of his birth.

In Japanese astrology, Jiro Murai is a fire dog. People born under that sign are absolutely charming, gentle and friendly, but they can get testy when pressured to do things that don't interest them. They love to party and their friends love their enthusiasm. They are artistic, honest and sincere, and they carry out whatever they undertake to do.

The preceding astrological description comes from the Internet, and as such needs to be taken with a grain of salt. Still, when I read that they "love to party" I couldn't help but think of Jiro Murai's wild ways as a youth, and of the many excesses that eventually led to the illness that was to change the direction his life took.

There was a time when physicians were also astrologers. Hippocrates (c. 460-356 B.C.), the father of medicine, laid the foundation for astrological typology. His theory of humors divided individuals into four temperament types: choleric, sanguine, phlegmatic, and melancholic. The human body is sensitive to its environment; we live and evolve in close connection with the universe.

Galen of Pergamon (129-c. 216), Nicolaus Copernicus (1473-1543), Paracelsus (1493-1541), and Nostradamus (1530-1566) all followed the path he had set. Samuel Hahnemann (1755-1843), the German physician who created homeopathy - that wretched doctor, as some called him - drew on Hippocrates' writings in developing his law of similitude. The American Andrew Taylor Still (1828-1917), the founder of osteopathy who devoted his entire life to the search for a different approach to healing that involved a fuller knowledge of ourselves, was interested in astrology, as was the Swiss psychoanalyst Carl Jung (1875-1961), to whom we owe the notion of the collective unconscious.

In the course of his research on Jin Shin Jyutsu, Jiro Murai studied Hippocrates, Pythagoras, and the Greeks in general. He was very familiar with Chinese moon-based astrology, and studied its various correspondences with Western sun-based astrology, and very likely with the Mayan calendar as well.[24]

In traditional Chinese medicine, there is a correlation between organs and planets. The rhythm of the Zodiac permeates everything. In Jin Shin Jyutsu, it is presented as the lumbar circle.

In *Jin Shin Jyutsu, Text II,* Mary Burmeister pairs each sign with an organ: Aries: lungs; Taurus: large intestine; Gemini: stomach; Cancer: spleen; Leo: heart; Virgo: small intestine; Libra: bladder; Scorpio: kidneys; Sagittarius: diaphragm; Capricorn: umbilicus; Aquarius: gall bladder; Pisces: liver.

The differences between signs matter less than their interpenetration. The twelve signs of the Zodiac co-exist in every individual. Life starts with Aries. We need its energy to come into the world and declare: "I AM!" There lies within us the various transformative phases of this energy as it passes from one sign to the next. And we need them all. When one of the phases becomes dominant, disharmony results.

The Japanese imported the Chinese Zodiac in the 7th century. The Sino-Japanese zodiacal cycle has twelve years, which corresponds to the time it takes Jupiter to complete its orbit around the sun.

Each sign is symbolized by an animal:

Ne (zumi) – Rat
Ushi – Ox
Tora – Tiger
U (sagi) – Rabbit (or Hare)
Tatsu – Dragon
Mi – Snake
Uma – Horse
Hitsuji – Sheep
Saru – Monkey
Tori – Rooster
Inu – Dog
I (noshishi) – Boar (or Pig)

The twelve signs combine with the five elements of the cosmos – earth, fire, metal, water, wood – to form a complete cycle of sixty years. The cycle begins with *Ki-no-E Ne* (wood, older brother, Rat) and always ends with *Mi-zu-no-To I* (water, younger brother, Pig). The terms "older brother" and "younger brother" are sometimes taken to be equivalent to "positive" and "negative." A person's cosmic element is determined by the last digit of the year of his or her birth:

Ka-ne (metal): 0 and 1
Mizu (water): 2 and 3
Ki (wood): 4 and 5
Hi (fire): 6 and 7
Tsuchi (earth): 8 and 9

The five elements represent the phases of a full cycle. The five-element theory, along with yin and yang, form the basis of Chinese medicine.

The *jikkan*, the ten-year cycle of the elements, and the *jyunishi*, the twelve-animal cycle, were used to measure time. Five cycles of twelve years corresponded to a lifetime. In ancient times, a span of twenty years represented one age in a person's life.

From birth to 20 years of age was childhood or youth. In Japan, the second Monday of January is coming-of-age day (*Seijin*), a holiday celebrating everyone who turned twenty.

From 20 to 40 is middle age, from 40 to 60, old age. *Kanreki* – the completion of the calendar – is a celebration held on a person's sixtieth birthday.

At 61, life begins anew.

Jin Shin Jyutsu tells the story of the transformation and densification of the vital life force, a process Mary Burmeister called "the study of the depths," with each depth corresponding to a specific age in a person's life: the first, from 0 to 15 years, the second, from 16 to 30, the third, from 31 to 45, the fourth, from 46 to 60, and the fifth, after 60. The sixth depth marks a return to the absence of form.

猫
Cat

The twelve animals of the cycle, called *jyunishi* (Earthly Branches), were not chosen randomly. Legend has it that when Buddha attained *parinirvana* upon his death, not only did throngs of followers attend the cremation, but animals did as well. The rat is said to have been the first to arrive, followed by the ox (or cow), the tiger, the rabbit (or hare), the dragon, the snake, the horse, the ram, the monkey, the rooster, the dog, and the boar (or pig). But no cats!

Cats hold a very special place in Buddhism. They are considered to be totally free spiritual beings endowed with clairvoyance and healing powers. In Japan, they are also considered good luck. *Maneki neko,* the beckoning cat, is a traditional figurine of a cat sitting on its haunches with its paw raised next to its ear. It is celebrated on September 29. In shops, it is customary to place a *maneki neko* by the door to beckon good fortune (with the left paw) and happiness (with the right) to come in.

Family Crest
Family Honor
Buried Treasure

It was 10:00 am, March 15, 2017 when Kyoko and I pushed open the door to City Hall in Daishoji, heading for the Civil Registry office. Japanese law requires every household to notify local authorities of births, marriages, divorces, and deaths. The information is inscribed in a family history called the *koseki*. Although the City Hall in Daishoji was a modern building, the large room housing the Civil Registry was heated by a simple oil-burning stove enclosed by protective wire fencing. A large gold-colored kettle sat on the stove, awaiting teatime. At window number 5, a charming clerk very carefully explained that because we were not family we could not have access to Jiro Murai's *koseki*.

Neither she nor any of the colleagues she discreetly consulted had heard of Jiro Murai or of Jin Shin Jyutsu. She did not know of any doctor Murai or any other Murais, for that matter. She suggested we try the public library.

Before World War II, it was not so much individuals as "houses," *ie* – generally speaking, households – that were recorded in the Civil Registry, and any given household could easily include more than twenty people: grand-parents, parents, brothers and sisters, uncles and aunts, and servants. Mention was made of the living as well as the dead, and even those not yet born. The household was the meeting ground for human beings and the kami each lineage worshipped. A misdeed committed by one family member sullied the honor of all of them. Everything was recorded in the *koseki* and stayed with the family "for all eternity." The head of the household had complete authority, but in return was expected to provide for everyone else. On the father's death, the position as well as all the family's possessions were passed on to the eldest son or, in the absence of a son, to the eldest daughter. Marriage served to maintain the lineage, to carry forward the cult of the family's ancestors, and to preserve the family's holdings. To assure the continuity of the family line, people often had to adopt. In addition to the main branch of the household there were the secondary branches of the second son or of a daughter whose husband the family had adopted; in the countryside, it was not uncommon for a secondary branch to be granted to a deserving tenant farmer.

In *The Life of Oharu*, Kenji Mizoguchi depicts the castes and households of feudal Japan. Oharu is the daughter of a nobleman, Okui Shinzaemon, a samurai of the Chion-In Temple. She is discovered in the arms of a boy from Lord Todo's household, Katsunosuke, who is of an inferior class. The prefect of Tokyo passes judgment on her sinful act, "Your position in the palace forbade involvement with a man of lower rank. You have broken the law. Such unspeakable behavior deserves exemplary punishment. You are to be banished from the capital, and your father and mother, who were responsible for your up-bringing and whose task it was to watch over you, will be cast out with you." The young man is summarily executed. The exiled young woman and her parents bid farewell to their family on a bridge and head off to the countryside. The father is furious with his daughter, but then luck comes knocking. Lord Matsudaira's wife is infertile. The lord is looking for a young woman who can bear him a child and perpetuate the family lineage. Oharu is chosen for her looks: no beauty marks, white teeth, a proper nose, and adequate space between her eyes. A doctor examines her and pronounces her fit to have children. She becomes a part of the lord's household only to be cast out penniless once she has given birth to an heir. Left to wander from house to house,

Oharu endures one ordeal after another until, utterly destitute, she is reduced to prostitution and begging.

Every household (*ie*) is associated with a family crest (*kamon*) that one often finds engraved on tombstones. The *mon* was originally a privilege of the aristocracy but was subsequently granted to warriors as well. By the 13th century, the privilege had been extended to all castes and served as a means of communication for a generally illiterate population. It was used to indicate an artisan's provenance, identify a trade or a shop, or the boundaries of property. Every household had a tombstone with its crest engraved upon it. The Murai gravesite we visited in the little cemetery near the Kayano Osugi cypress trees was thus clear proof that a Murai household had once lived nearby. And the Buddhist ornamentation we found on the gravestone is a reminder that medicine had long been the province of religion.

Before the Meiji Era, Japanese society was structured by a system of castes. At the top of the hierarchy were the warriors: shoguns, samurai, and their families. Then came the people who provided what was needed to live, the farmers, and further down those who transformed matter, the artisans. Merchants were near the bottom, for money was considered to be tainted… in principle, at least. At the margins were the outcasts, the *burakumin*, who included all tradesmen dealing in death: butchers, tanners, undertakers… A person born a *burakumin* had little chance, if any, to move up. Even more peripheral were the untouchables, the *hinin*, or non-humans: criminals and beggars. They, however, could re-integrate society.

Kenji Mizoguchi's *Tales of Ugetsu* is set in the 16th century, with the action taking place near Lake Biwa. An ongoing war provides two ambitious villagers with the chance to change their social status. One becomes a wealthy lord by marrying a ghost, the other a prestigious samurai by killing a lord's archenemy. But it is not in the nature of things to change castes, and their actions are not without consequence for their families. The first man's wife is murdered, the second man's wife ends up a prostitute. Through journeys between the visible and the invisible the two men eventually come to see the true meaning of their lives.

Families also lived together because they performed the same work. Traditionally, each family was associated with a specific trade or profession. The Murais were a family of physicians.

During the Edo period (1603-1868), the social status of doctors was a highly regarded intellectual calling and attracted people from all social backgrounds, especially samurai.

Japan had closed itself to the world for two centuries when, not long before Jiro Murai's birth, Commodore Perry and his notorious "Black Ships" forced the doors open. On July 8, 1853 four steamers – the *Mississippi*, the *Plymouth*, the *Saratoga*, and the *Susquehanna* – dropped anchor in Edo (Tokyo) Bay. Perry carried a message from President Fillmore enjoining the Japanese authorities to abide by the laws of international commerce. Japan complied.

Quickly realizing how far they had fallen behind economically, the Japanese threw themselves into a quest for progress. Railroads soon crisscrossed the entire archipelago, lighthouses blinked and flashed along the coast, a postal service emerged, and school became mandatory. The capital was moved from Kyoto to Edo and given the name Tokyo. In 1868, the Emperor, Prince Mutsuhito, who ushered in the Meiji era, declared, "For the salvation of the Empire, we must seek out Knowledge wherever it lies."

The long line of physicians in the Murai family were proponents of science-based medicine, but Jiro, the second son with the paradoxical personality, swam against the tide. While the rest of his family sought to free themselves from tradition and raced headlong towards a Westernized future – a loss of identity depicted in the writings of Yukio Mishima – Jiro Murai dedicated his life to the search for "treasures" buried in ancestral wisdom that could provide the tools with which people could help themselves.

In Japanese, two is *ni*.
Two / the second …
Double / Ever-changing

二
Two

The number two signals ambivalence and duality; it is the ultimate divider. In Chinese philosophy, dualism is expressed through yin and yang, which are inseparable. They refer to the bright and dark in all things, the negative and the positive, the feminine and the masculine, the terrestrial and the celestial. They represent opposites but that are never fully in opposition to each other, for the ever-present movement between them creates continuity. All things are now yin, now yang. This oscillation is the source of movement and gives the world its rhythm and dynamism. The Japanese *jikkan* and *Jyunishi* correspond to the Chinese yin and yang.

Kyoko asked me if the number 2 had particular meaning in Jin Shin Jyutsu.

Jiro Murai identified twenty-six specific areas in the body, which Mary Burmeister called "safety energy locks." Each is designated by a carefully chosen number between 1 and 26, and to master Jin Shin Jyutsu is to acquire knowledge of them. The number 26 means "complete," the state of Being in which we are fully present in the moment.

Safety energy lock number 2 is located in the lower back, at the tips of the left and right iliac crests of the pelvis. In the *Tao Te Ching* we read, "One begot two. Two begot three. And three begot the ten thousand things." Safety energy lock number 1, located on the medial side of the knee, deals with breathing out, number 2 with breathing in. The number 3 initiates movement. Safety energy lock number 2 is associated with the life force within all creatures, and with wisdom.

To alleviate discomfort in the back, to improve respiration or digestion, one need only place one's hands on safety energy lock 2 on the right and left rear side of the pelvis, which is what people often do instinctively when they are fatigued.

Back at the hotel, I found an email from my older brother. I, too, am the second born, a middle child with a younger and an older brother. Patrick is a micro-traveler. He has been exploring France for years, on foot, on horseback, on a sailboat, meticulously attentive to the tiniest details, the most minute changes. This is what he wrote that day, "Thank you for the news from Japan. The last news I had dated back to Nicolas Bouvier's two long stays there in the 1960s, during which one of his children was born. Bouvier described the extraordinary civility of the Japanese which, if you were not careful, could easily get you into trouble or at least make things extremely awkward."

The traveler-writer Nicolas Bouvier is also known for his translation of Basho's diary, which Basho wrote during his five-month, 1,500-mile trek from Kyoto up to the prefecture of Ishikawa, where Kyoko and I were now staying. In 1689, in *The*

Narrow Road to the Deep North, Basho wrote, "Whether we spend our lives sailing or watching our hair turn grey while driving a horse-drawn carriage, life itself is a journey, and the journey is home."[25]

Ancestors' names
Wells and Villages
Kanji

Provincial towns have the same feel everywhere. No one country or age has a monopoly on the boredom that pervades their streets. At the library – a modern building next to the Kutani Porcelain Art Museum – a Mrs. Shimizu received us with umpteen bows. Much to our surprise, she was expecting us. City Hall had called ahead to let the library know we were on our way and a staff member had been promptly assigned to deal with the foreigner and her acolyte. It was all so wonderfully considerate.

Mrs. Shimizu was a short, stout woman with a blue smock snuggly tied around her waist. She was delighted to be assisting us and already had thought about ways she might help. She quickly steered us to a section of books on the region. As we moved among the stacks, Kyoko whispered in my ear that Shimizu was her sister's married name. We took it as a sign! Another one was soon to follow: with obvious joy, Kyoko picked a book by Hiroshi Takada off the shelves and then learned from Mrs. Shimizu that this great friend of her mother's, the author of a well-known series of books on cats and essays on snow and fine Japanese paper, had lived in the area.

Mrs. Shimizu spread a few books out on a table. Some were written by the former mayor's father, others by a doctor whose grandson was still practicing in a local clinic. That was more than enough to keep our search going. The number of doctors was impressive (the French are writers, the Italians, architects, and the Japanese, doctors). When we learned that there was a physicians' district on the edge of town, I immediately conjured images of Jiro Murai spending his childhood there. Kyoko leafed through the phone book, searching for a Murai. She came across a Kumiko Murai, but we were not able to reach her.

Every time in the course of my quest that I thought I had shed light on some obscure area, three other mysteries would present themselves, so you can imagine how happy I was when I discovered that *murai* meant "village."

Had Jiro Murai written his Jin Shin Jyutsu manual for an entire village – the wealthy and the poor alike, the learned and the uneducated, the young and the old – in the hopes that every villager would learn how to perform it on himself like some daily self-care practice, or, if necessary, to treat an illness?

A village, *mura*, is the smallest incorporated district in Japan.

Murai – pronounced 'mula-E' – is written with two kanji, the second of which means "well." How could there be a village if there wasn't a well providing access to a source of water? I felt a thrill when I learned that *i* also meant "doctor." *Mura-i*, the village doctor. It sounded almost too good to be true! As it turned out, that *i* actually corresponds to a different kanji.

Chinese characters (Japanese kanji) first appeared in China in the 16th century B.C.E. They were originally pictograms or stylized drawings representing what people were trying to say. When they arrived in Japan in the 4th century C.E. there was no written form of language. The Japanese appropriated them immediately. According to legend, before their introduction the Japanese communicated by sending little stones to each other. A heart shaped stone meant, "I love you," a smooth, white one, "everything is fine," a rough stone, "things are tough."

A respectable Japanese dictionary lists more than four thousand kanji. After World War II, in an attempt to simplify matters, the government selected the 1850 most frequently recurring kanji, to which was added a separate list of 284 kanji used for first and last names.

On September 19, 1870, the Meiji Supreme Council granted the entire Japanese population the right to have a family name, regardless of caste or class. Five years later, the right became an obligation, "From this day forward, everyone must have a family name. Anyone who does not know the name of his ancestors will have to invent one."

Until that time, having a family name, like bearing arms, was a privilege reserved for the highest castes of noblemen and warriors. A high-ranking warrior would be announced with the name of his fiefdom, followed by the name of his castle, followed by the name of his clan and his court, and then his real name. In the *Kojiki* we find, "The Superior-Master-of-the-great-province,"[26] who also goes by Possessor-of-the-Great-Name, Superior-of-Plain-of-Reeds, Superior-Eight-Thousand-Spears, and Spirit-of-the-Country-of-Life. Five names in all. On a shrine register, a farmer would put down the name of his village followed by his personal name or nickname. A shopkeeper or an artisan might write down the name of his trade or his commerce. In Japanese movies, children call one another older brother, little sister, and so on.

A commoner did not have the right to a family name and was referred to in multiple ways:

The name of the household (*ie*) or the branch (*myoji*) he belonged to.

His birth name, which he lost after the coming-of-age ceremony (*genpuku*).

His real name (*imina*). This was a sort of secret identity never used except in official ceremonies, or perhaps in intimate moments between lovers.

His formal name, which was also given to him in childhood.

His everyday name, used by strangers.

His nickname, chosen by another person.

His assumed name. Whereas all of a person's other names

were given to him by someone else, this one he chose. To be sure, artists and intellectuals used assumed names more than other people.

His posthumous name.

All these names resonated differently at different times in a person's life, and even beyond death. They spun around him like a spiral around its axis, like the energy spiraling inside the body, from the skin to the bones.

In Japan, a name is not just a story; it is a saga.

The Meiji era that brought Japan out of its isolation and opened its doors to foreign influence was responsible for extraordinary social and cultural change. Commoners who were now required to have a family name took those of nobles, or used place names, or names that indicated their trade. Almost eighty percent of these names had some connection with nature.

Among the most frequent family names, I found the following:

渡辺

Watanabe (ferryman) as in Watanabe Kyoko and Watanabe Kazan (1793-1841), a painter and samurai. It is the 5th most common family name.

加藤

Kato (wisteria), as in Kato Haruki, Jiro Murai's disciple, Kato Sadaki, his son, Kato the kimono seller, and Shuson Kato, the poet. It is the 11th most common name.

村井

Murai, as in Murai Jiro, is 338th on the list. Where does the name come from? Did the Murai family belong to a privileged caste or did it claim the name in 1875? Could Jiro Murai be his nom de plume?

I shared this conjecture with Gaku Kondo when he came to visit. He himself was from a line of doctors and samurai. He told me that his own mother had inherited her uncle's family name and that she had given it to her husband and children. I expressed surprise.

"You mean your father just gave up his name?"

"That's right," Gaku said. "He had seven brothers and sisters. It wasn't a problem."

"How does that actually work?"

"You go to City Hall and ask to have the name changed in the koseki."

Of course! The famous register where everything is recorded.

As I was exploring the archives of samurai on the Internet I came across a Murai Sadakatsu (1547-1582) who served under Oda Nobunaga. This was the famous lord of the Oda clan who undertook the unification of Japan and who appointed Murai chief administrator of Kyoto in 1573. The territory of the Oda clan stretched all the way to Kaga.

I also discovered that under the Tokugawa shogunate (1603-1868) doctors, as well as scholars and Shinto priests, were allowed to use a family name even if they were not samurai.

雨

The Rain

It was pouring, a real torrential rain.

A Japanese kind of rain.

In Japanese films, the rain is a character.

For example, in Akira Kurosawa's *Rashomon*. Three men – a woodcutter, a priest, and a commoner – seek refuge from a downpour in the ruins of the old Rash-O-Mon portico in the ancient city of Kyoto. The woodcutter presents four versions of the same crime: the wife's version, the presumed murderer's version, the victim's ghost's version, and his own. Ryunosuke Akutagawa (1892-1927), the author of the short story "Rashomon" (1915) the film is based on, was effectively raising the question of what reality is. What is real?

On a first level lies the physical reality of the facts, actions, and words related to the "crime."

On a second, physiological level, lies the sensorial reality of the perception of sounds and light.

The third level is psychological, the imagined reality of meanings and values.

The fourth level is symbolic, the cultural reality of moral and religious principles.

Thus the same crime could be recounted, transformed, and re-interpreted through each witness' level of consciousness.

Similarly, each journey into Jin Shin Jyutsu is peculiar to the individual who embarks upon it, and totally dependent on that individual's level of consciousness.

To be conscious is to be open to what is happening in the present moment. "There is no such thing as a mistake," Mary Burmeister liked to say. "There is only what we experience. If anyone is to be forgiven, it is ourselves."

Birds Singing
Porcelain and Pastry
Precautions

The rain hadn't let up.

"It rains in my heart / As it rains on the town." Could the French poet Verlaine have been Japanese?

In Japanese, you don't say, "I miss you," but rather, "without your presence there is sadness."

Kyoko took me to the cafeteria in the Kutani Porcelain Art Museum. In France, the word "cafeteria" evokes a noisy room with tables strewn with the remains of previous patrons' meals. There was none of that there, only silence, harmony, and beauty. The atmosphere accorded perfectly with the Zen garden I could see outside. A fellow who must have emptied an entire shelf had spread out books on a nearby table and was busily studying them. I got the feeling that he was preparing a trip. A woman in a kimono, straight out of a Japanese print, glided over to our table and took our order, bowing with each word. She came back a little later with pastries and a lovely tea service on lacquered wooden trays, all of it so elegant it looked like a painting. In Japan, you do not drink tea in cups with handles, but in little bowls you hold with both hands, one beneath for support, the other on the side. As I picked up a bit of red bean paste with my chopsticks, I thought of Kyoko's friend, Misako Nemoto, whom I met the first day of my visit, and what she had to say about tastes, "The first time I came to Paris, I was nostalgic for fluffy, sweet cream pastries, for soft, delicate smoked chestnuts, for ice cream made with milk rather than cream or vanilla, and preserved mandarins as succulent and tart as in a dream. The gap between cultures seems particularly unbridgeable with regard to sweets. It is often harder to get used to desserts in another culture than to savory dishes."

I totally agree. I love Japanese food, but I gladly skip desserts. I cannot imagine being nostalgic for them. That said, I got so used to the seaweed candies we would get at the train station that I brought some back home with me.

トイレ
Toilets

Before leaving the museum we used the restrooms. I am always a little reluctant to go to a public bathroom, and when I am with a friend I seek a spot as far away as possible. Here, however, I was able to relax as I relieved myself, with the sounds I was making muffled by the singing of birds. Kyoko told me that the Japanese are constantly emptying their bladders, even if there is no need to, just as a simple precaution. In her house, as in most, there is a high-tech toilet with a heated seat and a spray for intimate hygiene. This is not consumer excess. There is no central heating in Japan; each room is heated separately. A heated toilet seat is hardly a luxury when the bathroom is ice cold in winter. The water spray helps prevent constipation and hemorrhoids.

Cleanliness has always been of tremendous importance in Japan, and *toire* (toilets) seem to have been used since the dawn of civilization. The first sewer systems date back to the Yayoi Period (300 B.C.E. to 250 C.E.). In 1585, in his *Treatise on the Contrasting Customs of the Japanese and Europeans,* Luis Frois noted this: "We put our privy outside, away from and behind houses. Theirs are in front, obvious, visible for all to see." "We sit down, they squat. In Europe, horse manure is spread in gardens and human waste is thrown into the gutter. In Japan, they throw horse manure in the gutter and nourish their gardens with human waste."[27]

In *In Praise of Shadows* (1933), Junichiro Tanizaki described these hallowed places thus: "It always stands apart from the house, at the end of a covered passageway, in a grove fragrant with leaves and moss. It is impossible to describe the sensation one feels as one squats in the dim light, basking in the faint glow filtering through the *shoji* (sliding screens), daydreaming or gazing out at the garden. The novelist Natsume Soseki (1867-1916) considered these morning trips to be one of life's great pleasures, albeit a purely physical one."[28]

In a place like this, Jiro Murai could meditate at leisure on the energetic function of the bladder.

In the course of his research, he discovered the existence of pathways of energy – known as flows – along which energy travels through our bodies like rivers. The three principal paths are the Main Central Energy, which flows through the center of the body, and the left and the right Supervisors that flow on either side. Together they form what is called the trinity flows.

There are also twelve organ flows, for the lungs, large intestine, stomach, spleen, heart, small intestine, bladder, kidneys, diaphragm, umbilicus, gall bladder, and liver.

To master the art of Jin Shin Jyutsu is to learn the pathways of our twelve "individualized" body function energies and how to stimulate them with the help of the universal life force.

Bladder function energy travels from the forehead to the little toe. It is a fourth-depth energy and it acts on the heart and the kidneys. Bladder function disharmony can lead to cystitis, incontinence, back pain, ear problems, or depression. In her self-help book, Mary Burmeister recommends harmonizing the bladder function energy as part of a daily routine, by placing one hand on the coccyx and the other behind the neck. The bladder function can also be stimulated by holding the index finger.

Kaga Onsen
The Physicians' District
Baths and Religion

We were headed for the physicians' district, making our way down the streets of Daishoji through a half-hearted mix of light rain, flurries, and fog. They say that the town was laid out so that each house would have a view of Mount Hakusan. I was wondering if the skies would ever clear and let us see it. Meanwhile, I took pictures of houses. Some were simple boxes of dark wood with potted plants for gardens and cube-shaped cars parked out front. Others were majestic homes with torii in the gardens, meticulously manicured grounds, and the kind of lovely, overhanging roofs you see on temples. There is nothing arbitrary about the way houses are oriented. Tradition has the entrance facing southeast, to receive all the positive energies, or directly south, toward the land of Buddha.

Under the awning of a big building with a zinc roof I noticed some strange looking vegetables hanging down from a bamboo rod: gigantic, oblong radishes. The Japanese love *daikon*. They chop it into thin slices that they add to their miso soup, simmer it with soy sauce, mix it in with their rice, or pickle it. And as with food of any kind, they are careful to point out its dietetic value: *daikon* is rich in vitamins, minerals, fibers, carotene, calcium and iron …

家
House

People are proud of this beautiful region and take pleasure in telling you so. The thermal baths date back to the 16th century.

The spring waters at Yamanaka Onsen, where Basho bathed, as did, most probably, Jiro Murai, are said to extend longevity. It is one of the three best hot springs in the country. Legend has it that 1,300 years ago a Buddhist monk who had come to hunt eagles was surprised to see a white heron (*shirasagi*) cleansing its injured leg in the stream. He concluded that the spring had magical powers, set people to work, and opened a thermal bath.

Between the men's and women's baths, under a mechanical clock in the square, stood a fountain beckoning passersby to come and drink. A sign listed the water's virtues, "Good for the gall bladder and rheumatism, helps prevent obesity." I loved to sit there around 6 p.m. and watch people come and go: women, children, older folk, folk not so old, some of them even young. After bathing, the men would join the women and chat for a while, after which they would ride off on their bikes. Kyoko told me that little children don't always like the baths. They are rewarded with fruit-flavored milk. She pointed out a tiny basin of thermal water in which eggs were cooked for breakfast.

I fondly remember the languorous hours I spent as a child in the warm mist of thermal baths as I concentrated all my energy on the simple task of breathing. Every summer, year after year, my parents would send me to La Bourboule, whose waters were known to help people with respiratory ailments like the asthma and chronic bronchitis I suffered from.

The healing virtues of mineral baths have been known to physicians for centuries, as far back as Hippocrates, Galen, and Paracelsus. The volcanic landscape of Japan features more than three thousand hot springs, some hidden deep in the mountains, others nestled along the coast. They are the primary tourist destination of the Japanese. The Portuguese merchant ship captain, Jorge Álvares, said the following in *Information about Things in Japan* (1548): "Their hot springs are thus: the water at the source of a wide stream is unbelievably cold, but further downstream, where the water is deep, it is just as unbelievably hot ... Winter and summer alike, I saw most of the women from the area wade into the stream or the sea before sunrise, dunk their heads three times and each time keep it underwater awhile, even when it was snowing. Then they slipped back into their clothes, filled wooden vessels with water, and walked through the streets sprinkling the water about with their fingers..."[29]

The traditional bath is a centuries-old Shinto practice of purification. People come not just to take care of their bodies but also to regenerate their spirit and purify their soul. Among the eight million divinities in Japanese mythology Mii-no-Kami is the kami of springs. At an *onsen*, people take three or four baths a day, as many as necessary until they feel stripped bare, totally cleansed of all ego and intention, and at a point where thought is no more. Now that I have experienced scrubbing my body from head to foot with ancestral ointments and balms like horse oil, coating my hair with the camellia oil sumo wrestlers use, sitting in a wooden tub with essential oils that improve circulation, feeling the texture of volcanic rock on the soles of my feet, and daydreaming in the fumaroles of an outdoor spring while gazing at the moon, I fully empathize with the Japanese who come to the West.

How do they survive without their baths?

The first Japanese doctor to prescribe therapeutic thermal baths was Goto Konzan (1659-1733), during the Edo period.

Because I suffered from asthma, I discovered how essential breathing was at a very early age. It also made me receptive to alternative medicines such as Jin Shin Jyutsu. In a work by Mieko Macé, *Médecins et médecine dans l'histoire du Japon (Physicians and Medical Practice in the History of Japan)*, I discovered that

Goto Konzan was also responsible for a *"Theory of the stagnation of the unique original breath"* (*Ikki Ryutai Ron*): "What I call the unique breath is that which shapes the human body: upper and lower, front and back, left and right, surface and depth. There is no area that this breath does not reach into and fill […] Once you understand that the stagnation of this unique breath is the cause of all illness, more than half your work is done."[30]

医
Doctor

According to every biographical sketch I had looked at, Jiro Murai was from a family of doctors and, according to some, a "prestigious" family of doctors. On that 15th of March, 2017, around 4 p.m., in between downpours and on the librarian's advice, we arrived at Dr. Kenzo Inasaka's clinic. On the way, we had had to take shelter in a news dealer's shop. The vendor, a bit past her prime and delighted at the coincidence, told us that she had been the doctor's patient for many years. Then, in mid-sentence, she abruptly turned and hurriedly shuffled off to the back room.

Had she gone to get a map?

Several minutes went by.

As we waited for her, we skimmed through the health magazines. Sadaki Kato had mentioned an article on Jin Shin Jyutsu that he thought might be useful when I met people, but the issue had not yet come out.

The woman finally reappeared. Japanese people are said to be very good at drawing, and I am convinced they are. I find it fascinating to watch Kyoko take notes. It takes great dexterity to draw kanji quickly, tiny little figures that seem to dance on the white of the page while our Roman script just blackens it with lines.

The vendor handed us a slip of paper.

Her drawing was indecipherable, so approximate and imprecise that Kyoko was dumbfounded, at a total loss for words. We literally ran out the door to keep from laughing, bowing as many times as we could.

Sunlight was filtering through the branches of a magnificent, one-hundred-and-fifty-year-old ginkgo standing in front of the clinic. The doctor would see us, the receptionist said. It did not happen often, but he had time between two patients... and perhaps a bit of curiosity. In our search for information about Jiro Murai, each time we arrived somewhere unannounced we were well received, whereas whenever we made the mistake of calling ahead we were turned away.

The clinic was bright and pleasant.

We met Dr. Inasaka upstairs, where he invited us into a small sitting area next to his office. I listened to Kyoko explain our reason for coming. Little by little I had started picking out words. I loved the intonation, the music, the cadence, the little guttural sounds, *sōōō* or *sōō*, *sōō* or *sō*, *sō*, *sō*, and *hai, hai* (yes, yes), *desné* (that's it), *so-desuka* (oh, really?). We couldn't have hoped for better. Dr. Inasaka was of the thirteenth generation in a line of doctors from the region. He and his family lived in the house he was born in. His great-grandfather, who planted the ginkgo, had run the Kaga medical center specializing in dermatology before Meiji (1875). His grandfather wrote the directory for the regional association of physicians. His father built the clinic.

The doctor went to fetch the directory. Kaga has always had a large number of doctors. Could that be because of the thermal baths? No, there is no connection! In Japan, thermal baths have no place in medical practice.

Doctor Inasaka came back with a large book that he leafed through in front of us.

He set it down on the table.

The words fell from his lips like a verdict.

Kyoko translated immediately.

No Murai.

Had I been able to read kanji I would have grabbed that book from his hands. I would have shamelessly transgressed all the rules of propriety. I would have looked to see if he wasn't making a mistake or hiding something from us. Had I been able to read kanji I would have looked to see with my own eyes if there really wasn't anyone named Murai on the list.

Modes of Medicine East and West *Kojiki*

Not a single Murai in the Kaga Physicians Directory. I couldn't get over it!

It was after this disappointment that I first heard the expression "Dutch medicine," and it wasn't until we left Kaga that I fully understood what it meant. I had heard the term a second time from Alexandre Leroi, who was writing a book on the subject, and yet again from Shinohara Ryuichi, the historian and former school principal who received us in the Daishoji Tourist Office.

蘭方	漢方
Ranpo Medicine	Kampo Medicine

Dutch medicine – Ranpo medicine – derives from the Western, science-based medicine that Dutch explorers brought to Japan at the end of the Edo period. It is the kind of medicine Kenzo Inasaka practices.

Between 1641 and 1853, Japan's isolationist policies drove foreigners out of the country. The lone exception was the Dutch, whose Dutch East India Company established a trading post on the island of Dejima in Nagasaki Bay. Alexandre Leroi wrote me the following, "The Dutch were confined to the fan-shaped, man-made island of Dejima and could directly address only the shogunate's official interpreters. But whereas they were deliberately denied access to Japanese knowledge and culture, the Japanese did what was necessary to satisfy their thirst for Western knowledge." *Rangaku*, or "Dutch Studies," was the analytical discipline that helped them grasp Western technology and medicine.

In 1774, the publication of the first Western work on anatomy to be translated into Japanese, *Kaitai Shinsho*, triggered fierce debates between partisans of traditional medicine and those drawn to the scientific precision of Western methods.

In *The Thousand Autumns of Jacob de Zoet*,[31] the novelist David Mitchell offers a description of life on Dejima at the beginning of the 19th century. He tells of the restrictions placed on the Dutch, their convoluted relationship with the shogunate through interpreters, and the training given to the first Japanese students of Western medicine.

In 1824, a German doctor associated with the Dutch community named Franz von Siebold opened a medical school with fifty students selected by the shogunate.

In 1838, Koan Ogata founded an institute for Dutch Studies, the *Tekijuku*, in Osaka.

In 1871, two German army surgeons, Drs. Hoffman and Mueller, were assigned the task of restructuring the medical curriculum and reorganizing Tokyo University.

In 1874, government guidelines for medical education and the creation of a national degree for physicians (*Isei*) heralded the end of professional studies in Kampo medicine. When these guidelines were implemented in 1884, medicine had effectively been institutionalized. By the end of the 19th century, the intellectual and progressive elite of Meiji society was essentially composed of Ranpo doctors.

The maternal grandfather of Haruki Kato, Sadaki Kato's father and Jiro Murai's heir, was a navy doctor who was first appointed head of the military hospital and then president of its medical school. He went to Paris at the beginning of the Meiji period to study at the Institut Pasteur. Could he have been part of the Kitasato team that developed the antitoxin serums for tetanus and diphtheria? Could he have crossed paths with Alexandre Yersin, the bacteriologist and explorer who isolated the bacillus responsible for the bubonic plague and who is the protagonist in Patrick Deville's *Plague and Cholera*?[32]

Haruki was born at seven months, at a time when incubators for premature babies did not exist. His health was fragile. Following hernia surgery, he developed chronic intestinal problems and did not walk. His parents were progressives attracted to the West. They sought the help of Ranpo doctors who proved unable to make a diagnosis and could not cure him. The family then turned to a fellow named Kurokawa, an acupuncturist and shiatsu Master who had been recommended to them. Haruki started walking just one week after treatment began, totally healed.[33] Haruki Kato writes of how his family suddenly started believing in the "mysterious" power of Oriental medicine, and how they subsequently encouraged him to study with Jiro Murai. The story is further indication of how Kampo, which had been the only kind of medicine for centuries, had by this time lost its place in the Japanese way of life.

Kyoko is familiar with Ranpo medicine but no other. As far as she knows, it is the only form of medicine practiced in Japan, with the possible exception of homeopathy. Both her grandfather, a physician, and her uncle, an otolaryngologist, trained in "Dutch medicine," which she calls "German medicine."

Kampo medicine, known simply as Kampo, evolved from Traditional Chinese Medicine (TCM). It flourished in Japan in the 9th century after adapting to the Japanese and to the archipelago's native plants. For a practitioner of Kampo medicine, a health issue is not an attack that calls for a riposte, but rather an indication that the harmony between *in* and *yoh* (yin and yang) has been lost and needs to be restored. Everything is classified under one of the five elements – wood, fire, earth, metal, and water –, to which are associated the four cardinal points, the four seasons, and changes in weather patterns. To make a diagnosis (*shoh*), a Kampo physician takes a patient's pulses, palpates the abdomen, and examines the patient's face.

Kampo medicine went into sharp decline at the end of the 19th century when the Meiji government made it mandatory for physicians to take exams on Western medicine. But the creation of the Japanese Society for Oriental Medicine (*Nihon Toyo Igakukai*) in the aftermath of World War II laid the foundation for a modern-day Kampo. Besides acupuncture and moxibustion (which one sees in Yasujiro Ozu's film *Floating Weeds* when a young woman uses moxa on a theater company director), Kampo treatments make use of dried or heated plant-based remedies (*Kampo yaku*), like roots, leaves, bark, flowers, fruit, and seeds, and even animal parts, such as skin and bone. Other treatments are mineral-based. The most popular plants are *kanzo* (licorice root) and *yohkyoh* (ginger).

Kyoko's cold was an excellent excuse for us to step into a Chinese pharmacy and admire roots of all sorts and an old mortar.

Prior to the Meiji era, medical degrees did not exist. Doctor status was passed on from father to son, and accredited by the shogunate. In 1585, Luis Frois observed, "In our country, a person who practices medicine without having passed the exam can be punished and barred from the profession. In Japan, just about anyone can earn a living as a doctor. Our doctors prescribe medicine to be bought at the apothecary's; in Japan, doctors give out homemade remedies. We still sew up wounds; they apply a sticky piece of paper to them. We practice blood-letting; they use small, smoldering lumps of herbs. For men and women alike, our doctors take the pulses first of the right arm, then of the left. In Japan they start with the left for men and the right for women."[34]

From the end of the 18th century to the beginning of the 20th, medical practices were at the heart of all the intellectual debates underlying the modernization of Japan.

Akira Kurosawa's *Red Beard* (1965) is set in 1820, in Koishikawa, a neighborhood of Edo, the former name of Tokyo. The film's dashing protagonist, Naboru Yasumoto, is a freshly minted graduate of a Dutch medical school in Nagasaki and a man with grand aspirations: he wants to be the shogun's personal physician. But his first assignment is to a rural clinic run by Dr. Kyojio Niide, Red-Beard, (undoubtedly an inside joke on Kurosawa's part, since this was the term commonly used in referring to the Dutch). The clinic offers shelter to the sick and sometimes their families, provides meals for them, and prepares its own medical compounds. A garden of medicinal plants and a ward for the mentally ill adjoin the main building, which includes treatment facilities and patients' rooms, but there are no tatamis, because the clinic cannot afford them. The arrogant Yasumoto quickly begins acting the rebel in the hopes of being dismissed. He refuses to put on a doctor's uniform and goads a young nymphomaniac. But when Red-Beard has him sit by a dying patient and observe the last moments of the man's life he is profoundly unsettled. He is gradually won over by the unique personality of his master and begins to understand that compassion is indispensable in the fight against poverty and ignorance. Knowledge is important, to be sure, but empathy is more important still. As he becomes aware of his responsibilities as a physician, Yasumoto calls into question his initial aspirations.

漢方
Traditional Chinese Medicine

Because medicine was part of Buddhist training, it was long the practice of monks. During the *Shengoku* period – the Age of Warring States – in the 16th century, samurai also trained in dressing wounds and in obstetrics. They were known as *kinso-i* (*kin*: "sword;" *so*: "wound;" *i*: "medicine") and were somewhat comparable to Europe's barber surgeons. The physicians employed by the shogunate and by various lords functioned as civil servants. They received an annuity, were required to shave their head like monks, and could pass their office on to their offspring. They stood outside the caste system. In the private sector, physicians belonged to the same class as artisans. They made a respectable living from their trade, carried a sword like samurai, and had the right to bear a family name.

The first medical school was founded in Kyoto by Manase Dosan (1507-1594) upon his return from his studies in China. He gave up his monk's robe and began training students of all backgrounds. His teachings included a code of deontology and rapidly spread throughout the archipelago. In his *Manual of the Practice of Medicine* (*Keiteki-shu,* 1574) he wrote, "Applying the principles of wise men while taking into consideration each patient's condition… that is what medicine is about…"[35] Of the sources available to us, the *Inner Canon of the Yellow Emperor* is the most ancient of the texts on Traditional Chinese Medicine. The Yellow Emperor is said to have lived between 2697 and 2598 B.C.E. His *Inner Canon* is a treatise on spiritual acupuncture that aims at re-establishing the harmony between man and nature by increasing or decreasing the circulation of yang energy and determining through observation the state of a patient's breathing and the nature of his breathing patterns.

As a complement to this thought, Nagoya Gen-i wrote in 1691, "Whoever wants to study medicine should read Confucius."[36]

In reading Anne Millerand's dissertation *La Modernisation de la médecine, d'Edo à Meiji, rupture ou continuité (The Modernization of Medicine from the Edo to the Meiji era: Rupture or Continuity),* I was moved when I came upon a description of the principles of Jin Shin Jyutsu. "At the end of the 16th century, the Confucian principle '*I-wa-Jin-Jyutsu*' ('Medicine is the art of true Virtue') made its way into the world of Japanese medicine. In Confucian terminology, Jin means benevolence, humanity, 'perfect Virtue,' or, in Confucius's words, 'having enough self-control to restore in one's heart the honesty it received from nature;' and Jyutsu means 'art.'" The idea had already been expressed in the 7th century by Sun Simiao (581-682), China's King of Medicine and author of the best-known work of the first millennium, *Bei Ji Qian Jin Yao Fang (Essential Formulas for Emergencies Worth a Thousand Pieces of Gold).* The place that Sun Simiao, a Daoist and Confucian philosopher, occupied in Asia was equivalent to that occupied by Hippocrates in the West.

仁神術
Jin Shin Jyutsu

Jiro Murai was born in the midst of the debates between the adepts of Ranpo and Kampo medicines. He was surely conversant with the knowledge found in both Chinese medicine and Confucianism. In Jin Shin Jyutsu, it is said that a good doctor treats the invisible. In choosing a name for his physio-philosophy, Jiro Murai hesitated between the art of benevolence, the art of happiness, and the art of longevity. He finally settled on three kanji: *jin* (virtue, compassion), *shin* (Creator, man), *jyutsu* (technique, art). In the West, this became "the Art of the Creator through man of knowing and compassion."

The official French, American, and German JSJ websites, (the three I can read) present Jin Shin Jyutsu as the art of harmonizing the life energy in the body, effectively borrowing Mary Iino Burmeister's words. We are told that it was born of ancient wisdom and passed down orally from generation to generation before gradually falling into oblivion. It is said that the keys to this "buried wisdom" can be found, in part, in the *Kojiki*.

The *Kojiki* is a compilation of poems, songs, and folk tales recited by Hieda-no-Are and written down by the chronicler O-no-Yasamuro. It was compiled at the Empress Gemmei's request and presented to her in 712. The text refers to Japan as the Middle Country of Reed Beds. It is connected to the Celestial Plain by the Floating Bridge of Heaven, and to the Shadowy Land of the Dead by the Slope down into the Land of Darkness.

Mieko Macé approached her research believing that shamanic healing practices had currency in ancient Japan, but after examining ancient texts she concluded that "strangely, the first works written in Japanese, *Records of Ancient Matters* (*Kojiki*, 712) and *Chronicles of Japan* (*Nihon Shoki*, 720) never directly allude to such practices. There rather emerges from the myths a very realistic vision of illness as inherent to the human condition, like death itself. The divinities of illness and healing are paired. Like defilement and purity, one is inconceivable without the other."[37]

Shintoism has neither a founding figure nor a sacred text, like the Buddhist Sutras or the Bible. The word *Shinto* (the way of the kami) first appeared in the 6th century when it became necessary to differentiate it from Buddhism. Shintoism is the spiritual dimension of a people sensitive to and believing in the forces of nature. It was so intrinsic a part of Japanese identity that it had no name. In *Aux sources du Japon: Le shinto* (*At the Sources of Japan: Shinto*), the oriental scholar Jean Herbert explains that "what characterizes Shintoism is the profound conviction that divinities (Kami), human beings, and all of nature are in fact born of the same ancestors and are thus related... When in the course of Creation solid matter appeared, two Kamis, *Izanagi* and *Izanami*, at once spouses and siblings, created the universe, both what we perceive and what escapes our perception." Jean Herbert also quotes the great 15th century Shintoist, Urabe-no-Kanetomo, "What resides in the universe is called *Kami*, what resides in all things is called spirit (*Tama*), and what resides in human beings is called heart (*Kokoro*)."[38] In Shintoism, the human and the divine are one.

Life is a unique force manifest in every organism: plants, animals and human beings alike. In Greece, this energy is called *pneuma*, in India *prana*, in China *chi*, and in Japan *ki*. The concept of vital energy permeating the entire universe and giving life to all things is not merely a philosophical belief. In traditional medicines (Chinese and Ayurvedic), it also provides a practical approach to life and to healing. To heal, we need to harmonize the flow of vital energy within us.

For Jiro Murai, the universe is a reflection of what we are, and we are made of the same stuff as the stars. Jin Shin Jyutsu is the art of awakening our awareness to this universal life energy and teaching us how to diffuse it into various parts of the body to restore harmony, the absence of which is the cause of most illness. Jiro Murai believed that human beings possess the tools with which to heal themselves: their hands and breath. Every one of us has the capacity to fight off pain and sickness. The essential and wonderful message of Jin Shin Jyutsu is that there lies within each of us a healer.

Jin Shin Jyutsu is about learning to know (help) oneself. Mary Burmeister was tempted to change the name of Jin Shin Jyutsu to "Now Know Myself." At one of her talks, she told a student: "If you ask me what you should study, I'll say to you: yourself. If after studying yourself you ask me what you should study next, I will say again: yourself."

Childhood
Floating World
Kendo

That evening, I was so tired that resisting the call of the futon seemed beyond me and I said I would probably skip the baths.

How in the world can anyone say such a thing!

Kyoko, who had spent the entire day holding my hand on the rickety suspension bridge spanning the abyss separating her language from mine, let go of me. She whispered to our host that I was exhausted and had decided against a bath. It was as if I had said, "I am starving; I'd rather not eat." At the bar, Yuko and the regulars pricked up their ears, eager to relish the moment. They purred, meowed, and cleared their throats.

I suddenly felt as if I had lost my footing.

I was adrift in a floating world of words, as Akira Mizubayashi put it in *Une langue venue d'ailleurs* (*A Language Come from Afar*).[39]

Pour me a glass of saké!

I wasn't about to make another mistake and pour one for myself.

A large glass of warm saké! Saké for the ladies!

No moon no flower
To drink his saké
There, he is, all alone

– Basho

I looked up at the screen. There was a baseball game on.

Japan was playing Israel, and had just scored. The man next to me grunted his delight. He was a baseball manager and his son was on the verge of becoming a star. Doctor Inasaka, whom we had met earlier that afternoon, was also a baseball fan.

Did Jiro Murai play baseball? Was he a kendo enthusiast or an archer? Baseball came to Japan in the 19th century via a path that remains unknown. It has been played in schools and universities since 1880. During the Meiji era, when enthusiasm for the West was rapidly taking hold, medicine and education, which reached into all levels of society, were major conduits for the profound changes Japanese society was undergoing. School was made mandatory, and it was there that children learned to play baseball, the sport of Japan's archenemy in World War II, as Doctor Inasaka noted. In 1868, when wearing a sword was outlawed and samurai were forced to cut off their topknots, they went to the West to study law and medicine. The martial arts had by then lost much of their popularity and underwent name changes. *Kenjutsu* became *kendo* (the way of the sword). It is an art that demands agility, self-control, and precision. It has become a competitive sport again and is required in middle schools. Sundays in Tokyo, I saw lots of children doing kendo in temple dojos. Kyoko started learning the art at fifteen. She spent the first few months of her training watching older children practice, fascinated by their movements and outfits. Similarly, archery (*yumi*) is now called *kyodo* (the way of the bow). The archer has to summon the essence of three qualities: truth (*shin*), Zen virtue, and beauty (*bi*).

There Was a Father.

Yasujiro Ozu's *There Was a Father* depicts the everyday life of a widower and his son back in the day when people found entertainment in watching trains go by. Father and son share a love for fishing. Three scenes at the river, each one showing the son at a different age, divide the film into parts. You see middle-schoolers wearing uniforms and caps similar to those I saw on trains and buses, taking school trips with their teachers, and having their picture taken, as tradition demands, in front of the

Great Buddha of Kamakura. The father takes his son to an *onsen* inn, and they go to the men's baths for a moment of male bonding. In the exclusively male middle school, the boys learn English, but they also spend time weeding the garden. When the father drops his son off, he gives him two kinds of medicine and tells him to keep his stomach warm. The father often spends time at a Go club and dreams of marrying his son to his friend's daughter. There is always a kettle on the brazier in his house, where people walk barefoot on tatamis and bow before an altar to their ancestors. Social interaction is very formal and filial affection barely comes through the flow of words. There is no touching. Yasujiro Ozu shows us life in its repetitive reality. It is as if what was most important to him was to capture all that is not shown or said. His favorite actor, Chishu Ryu, bears a physical resemblance to Murai.

Here in Kaga, which had a different name when Jiro Murai was alive, life between the mountains and the sea has always been rather peaceful. Every neighborhood has a name: the Linen Fields district, the Fish district, the Archery district, the Smiths' district, the Eagle Keepers' district... this last one an indication of the presence at some point of lords and a castle. Originally, it was a rather poor region, known for the excellent quality of its rice, probably because rice was so difficult to grow here and required great care and effort. When you hear Kaga, Kyoko told me, you think *koku*, a unit of roughly 330 pounds (150 kilos), which, historically, was considered the amount needed to feed one person for a year, and which was used to measure a lord's wealth. Towards the end of the Edo period, the shogunate was collecting nearly six million of the national production of about 256 million koku. During the Meiji era the koku was replaced by the metric system. In 1585, Luis Frois noted, "Whole wheat bread is our food staple; for the Japanese, it is unsalted rice."[40]

Kaga is in the North, where the climate is harsh. Children make a game of guessing the next day's weather by throwing their wooden clogs (*geta*) into the air. If a clog lands upside down, it is going to rain. The Japanese have a profound sense of the seasons. Before the Gregorian calendar was adopted during the Meiji era they used the Chinese calendar. The Chinese have the same seasons we have, but with different dates. Whereas the solstices and equinoxes mark the beginning of the seasons in the West, the Chinese consider them to be peak moments, the essence of seasons, and therefore place them in the middle. Each season lasts about ninety days and has its period of emergence, its apex (the solstice or the equinox), and its period of decline.

Besides spring, summer, fall, and winter, Chinese tradition recognizes a fifth season, which mirrors the five-element theory. During this in-between season, which lasts 15 – 20 days, the weather anticipates the imminent transformation of energy: from January 18 to February 4, the coming of spring; from April 19 to May 6, the coming of summer; from July 22 to August 8, fall; October 22 to November 8, winter. These periods are associated with the color yellow and are a time in which to reestablish the yin-yang balance. The transitions from one season to the next explain why the five elements are represented in a specific order, in a circle in which Earth is located between summer and fall, which gives the sequence: wood, fire, earth, metal, and water.

The human body, which long ago was thought to be a microcosm subject to the same laws as the macrocosm of nature, has to adapt to the change of seasons. Allergies, colds, coughs, and ear, nose, and throat ailments are frequent as we transition into winter or summer, when eighty percent of the Japanese take the precaution of wearing masks. Kyoko does not wear one, but she learned at an early age that in addition to washing her hands, she had to gargle when she returned home from a trip to the city.

The sound of someone
Blowing his nose in his fingers
Plum trees in bloom

– *Basho*

Dr. Inasaka told us that sixty years ago there were no baths in private homes. To cleanse themselves, people went to public baths or the river. Soap, he pointed out, does not lather is sea-water. Yojiro Takita's magnificent film *Departures* includes several beautiful bath scenes that show us how very sensitive the Japanese are to the softness of water. People heated their homes with wood fires, drank well water, and ate fish, rice, and locally grown vegetables. An earthquake that killed thirty people made a deep impression on the doctor when he was eight years old. Winters, when it snowed, which it did more often when he was a young man than it does now, he would go skiing, and he also practiced meditation and read a lot. He recommended Kenji Miyazawa's *Night on the Galactic Railroad,* a fantasy novel written in 1927 about children traveling into the Beyond. The mantle of silence cast by a snowfall invites contemplation and haiku writing. Composing poetry is a widespread tradition in Japan. It is a sign that one is cultured, and was encouraged by Emperor Meiji whose Poetry Bureau, in what was to become a tradition, would every year choose a theme on which poetry lovers were invited to submit a 31-syllable tanka (5-7-5-7-7). Thousands of poems would come in, and thirty of them would be read to the Imperial family. You can read all these anonymously written haiku in the Basho museum in Yamanaka, a converted old inn with lacquered beams. Dr. Inasaka told us that the Kaga region, which once had a printing works, is known for its writers. His family was well-off and the physicians in the district held each other in mutual respect. His father was forty-three when he was born, and his grandfather, the doctor-writer, fifty-one when his own son, Dr. Inasaka's father, was born.

Kenzo spoke to us about a ceremony (*gongan shinji*) that takes place in February. Half-naked men pound bamboo shafts into pieces to make a braided rope representing a snake and throw it into the sea. I still don't know what this ritual is supposed to mark. Japan is the country with the greatest number of observances. There is always somebody's memory to honor, some ritual to carry out. People go to temples and shrines as easily as they drop in on friends. Respect for rituals is a poetic way of being part of the community, of wearing one's kimono, and so on.

Bonzes and morning glories
Reincarnated, how many times?
Long live the old pine tree

– *Basho*

These observances, which occur on every calendar day, seem to respond to a need to fully embrace the present moment and weave together all the nuances of human life as it unfolds, while keeping our lives in constant contact with the goddess Amaterasu, the Sun. In Japan, there is a god for everything, for every stage of life and every moment. I actually brought back with me the statue of a god that protects old people from falling in the bathroom.

Jin Shin Jyutsu also relates the changes of the seasons and the planets, and the way they interact with each other through the six depths defined by Mary Burmeister, which constitute the energetic blueprint of our lives. In our life's journey, the first depth represents arrival. During our first fifteen years Saturn helps define the contours of our bodies. The more solidly constituted one is at this first depth, the greater a person's sense of security, and the freer he or she will be to relate to the world under the influence of Venus, at the second depth, when, from 16 to 30, people develop their sensibility and ideals. The third depth, from 31 to 45, under the aegis of Jupiter, is that of a person's growth and fulfillment. The fourth depth covers mid-life, the years from 46 to 60, when, accompanied by Mercury, a person narrows the paths he or she wishes to continue to pursue. Beginning at 60, at the fifth depth, people who have made the right choices have nothing left to prove; they can simply shine with Mars. At the sixth depth, with the Moon, we prepare to gracefully negotiate the end of physical life.

The six depths correspond to six domains and constitute a classification that encompasses all things, from the most insubstantial to the densest. The first depth corresponds to the epidermis that delineates the body. At the second depth, connective tissue weaves together the different layers of the body. At the third depth, blood and fluids diffuse microscopic biochemical information throughout the body, connecting all parts. At the fourth depth, muscles initiate movement. At the fifth, bones allow for the body's posture. At the sixth, the body is perfectly balanced.

Jin Shin Jyutsu illustrates this narrative with a six-pointed star, with the six planets reflecting the sun that shines in the middle and which symbolizes the seventh depth and universal energy.

Spring, Summer
Celebrations and Traditions
Numbers

Jiro Murai had a turbulent youth. He liked to party and loved his fun. In Marseille, one day, I was trying to imagine what his life must have been like when I came upon Louis Frédéric's wonderful *Fêtes et traditions au pays du Soleil levant* (*Celebrations and Traditions in the Land of the Rising Sun*)[41] at a used-book stall. I found out that there are not many days in Japan without some secular or religious ceremony, some holiday or commemoration. These observances mark out the year and connect the Japanese to the land of their ancestors, to its myths and legends, and to their profound relationship with nature as well. And the dates of these observances constitute a language rich in symbols and secret meanings that very likely inspired Murai when he named the twenty-six safety energy locks. For example, contrary to Western tradition, 13 is considered lucky, and on March 13 all thirteen-year-olds celebrate their birthday in a temple. On the other hand, the word *shi*, which can mean both "four" and "death," is never to be pronounced on the New Year, and the fourth day of the month is considered unlucky.

In Jin Shin Jyutsu, numbers are a veritable language. Safety energy lock 13 is located in the chest, between the heart and the lungs, and its number evokes creative energy, regeneration, giving birth, and the desire for that which has not yet come into being. Safety energy lock 4 is located at the base of the skull on either side of the occipital ridge. The number suggests a window, a passage between energy and matter, a bridge between life and death. You place your hands on energy lock 4 to help someone who is pregnant, or help a dying person let go.

Given his joyful disposition, it is highly likely that as a little boy Jiro loved these celebrations, beginning with those of the *Shogatsu* for the New Year, the most important ones on the Japanese calendar. The Murais' house would have been decked out and had flowers displayed in their *tokonoma*. All the delicacies served that day would have been selected to bring good fortune: sweet potatoes, to bring wealth; daikon to bring a stable and successful life symbolized by this vegetable's deep roots; black soybeans, called *kuro mame*, to ward off bad spirits; and sea bream, because it is the king of all fish. And all of these foods would be accompanied, naturally, by a considerable number of cups of saké. (The Japanese are usually merry when inebriated.) The entire family would have awakened early to watch the first sunrise of the year and to honor the goddess Amaterasu, before donning their formal kimonos and proceeding to the Shinto shrine to pay their first visit of the year.

The Murai children would have received gifts, flown kites, or played *sugoroku* (Snakes and Ladders). On January 2, Jiro would have practiced his *kakizome*, the first calligraphy of the year, writing kanji that bode well.

Fallen to the ground
The kite
Soulless

– *Kubota*[42]

January 7 is the Festival of the Seven Herbs (*Nanakusa-no-Sekku*), an ancient Chinese tradition brought to Japan during the Heian period (794-1185). On that day, people eat a rice porridge called *kayu*, flavored with the seven wild herbs that are the first to appear in winter. The dish is known for its ability to purge the body of impurities, which is much welcome after the excesses of New Year celebrations. The day before, the herbs are laid out on a cutting board and pointed in the direction of good luck that year, alongside seven traditional cooking utensils, among them a rice scoop, a mortar and pestle, chopsticks, and a grater. The herbs are then finely chopped while people intone a traditional song that translates approximately, "Before the birds of the continent fly off toward Japan, let us receive the seven herbs of spring."

The second Monday of January is *Seijin Shiki*, a coming of age ceremony for everyone who turned twenty the previous year. Jiro would have put on his kimono and gone to the temple or to city hall. The ceremony marks the end of youth and the transition into adulthood.

Mid-January is the time of *Nyugaku Shiken*, entrance exams for schools at all levels.

It is also the time of sumo tournaments. Sumo is a national sport, a somewhat religious form of wrestling that is quintessentially Japanese. In former times, matches took place on the grounds of Shinto temples. The combatants are huge men often weighing more than three hundred pounds. They begin by throwing salt into the ring to purify it, after which they stomp the ground heavily with one foot and then the other to crush the forces of evil. The referee is dressed like a Shinto priest and is usually a member of a distinguished family. The young adepts who attend sumo schools must abide by an extremely rigorous regimen and go through grueling training sessions. It is impossible to turn on the television in Japan without coming across a sumo match.

春
Spring

Our February 3 and 4 used to be the beginning of spring on the Chinese calendar. Spring is associated with the color green and ascending movement. It is the beginning of the yang phase of the year.

On the day of *Setsubun* (division between seasons), throngs used to crowd temples to watch demons being expelled. Monks, priests, public figures, and sumo wrestlers would throw soybeans to the crowd and yell, *"Oni-wa soto! Fuku-wa-uchi!"* ("Get out, demons! Good fortune, come in!"). Shinto tradition does not believe in the notions of good and evil. Any phenomenon can be good or bad, depending on circumstances. That said, some kami, called oni, are more malevolent than others and can be responsible for deadly diseases.

The old pond
A frog jumps in
The sound of water

– Basho

March 3, the third day of the third month, is *Hina Matsuri*, Dolls' Day, also known as Girls' Day. It dates back to the Heian period when dolls bore the image of important figures at the imperial court and were supposed to be a protection against evil spirits. Did Jiro have sisters? If so, the collection of dolls inherited from previous generations would have been on display in his house. Kyoko's 18th century dolls are splendid in their silk attire. She inherited them from her father's family, one of whose ancestors was part of the imperial court. On Dolls' Day, the little girls in Jiro's family would have eaten on dishes from a doll set.

A day for young girls
Figurines of the Emperor
Long may he reign!

– *Basho*

On March 13, for his thirteenth birthday, Jiro would have put on a formal kimono to go with his family to a temple or shrine. It was originally a Buddhist ritual in which parents prayed to Kokuzo Bosatsu to grant their children protection, wisdom, and intelligence. In a country so vulnerable to natural catastrophes, life is ever entwined with the notion of chance, both good fortune and bad.

O-higan, the Day of the Dead, falls mid-March. Buddhists believe this to be the time when Buddha guides the souls of the dead towards nirvana. People go to cemeteries, burn incense, and place flowers on graves. In Kiyoshi Kurosawa's (not to be confused with Akira Kurosawa) *Journey to the Shore,* Yasuke takes his wife Mizuki on a journey through villages and rice paddies to meet the beings who helped him locate her after he died three years before, drowned and lost at sea. The day I left Tokyo, Kyoko and I said good-bye at the Shinjuku train station. I was headed for Narita airport, while she was leaving for Gotenba, near Mount Fuji, to pay homage to her mother at her gravesite. "*O-higan* is our All-Saints-Day," my friend explained. "It means 'the other quay, the other bank.' We bring flowers, burn incense, and purify gravesites. There are two *O-higans* a year, one at each equinox, spring and fall. On *O-higan,* she said, we visit our loved ones, whereas on *O-bon,* which is in the summer, their spirits come home. I never come to France before mid-August because there is no way I would miss *O-bon,* when the whole family gets together in Kyoto."
When Kyoko's friend Misako Nemoto, a professor and writer, spoke to me about *O-Higan,* she revealed that her father had the

kanji "universe" inscribed on his tombstone. The kanji represents the Shintoist notion that human beings are but one element in a vast universe.

Hanami, "Flower Viewing," is celebrated in late March or early April. Day after day, the weatherman informs people about where the cherry blossoms will be at their peak, from the South up through the entire archipelago to the North. It would be hard for anyone who has not experienced the unforgettable magic of the light blending into the whiteness of the flowers to imagine what it is like. There are cherry trees everywhere in Tokyo, lining avenues, in parks, and in cemeteries. Lanterns are hung from their branches. Are they beginning to bloom? Partially in bloom? In full bloom? I learned to distinguish about eighty per cent of the blooming phases.

Tomorrow, the cherry blossoms in Tokyo's Ueno district will surely have reached their peak. Everybody will be out in the street – students, employees, and families. They will unfold mats under the trees, take their shoes off and arrange them neatly, and celebrate the joy of the ephemeral. Emotions will be stirred when a breath of wind scatters the petals. People will sing and drink saké. People in love will declare their feelings. When after a few days, tiny beads of green begin to pierce through the stunning white, people will be so overcome with nostalgia that they will just want to hop on a train and head north.

In Kumano, the cherry trees illuminate the dark hillsides with pallid swaths of white. In Kaga, cherry trees line the river, and people drift downstream in boats beneath an archway of flowers. At night, before stopping on a bridge to experience *Hanami* one last time and pop the cork on a bottle of white wine, they peek through the dazzling branches to get a glimpse of the moon. In Kanazawa, they are feeling a bit tipsy. They lean against the trunk of a gnarled centenarian tree, give it a hug, and inhale the scent of the bark. And they stay there a long while, gazing at just one bough, or branch, or flower whose image they will treasure in their hearts until the next year.

First cherry blossoms
To see them extends my life
Seventy-five years

– *Basho*

School starts in April.

Japanese schools promote group cohesion. Young Hatsune, who came to visit us with his parents, told us that the school principal assembled all the students several times a week to lecture them. In Hiroshima, I saw a group of middle-schoolers on a trip with their teacher. The children were repeating his words in unison. "What we have seen here and what we have felt here we will never forget. We will create a peaceful world and bring peace everywhere." Keisuke Kinoshita's film *Twenty-Four Eyes*, adapted from Sakae Tsuboi's novel, chronicles the period from the late 1920s to Japan's post-war period. In the opening scene, a group of adorable little seven- or eight-year-olds in kimonos and rice straw sandals are on their way to pay a visit to a teacher recovering from an accident.

夏
Summer

According to the Chinese calendar, summer begins on May 6. It corresponds to the color red and centrifugal movement. It is the apex of the yang phase of the year.

The fifth day of the fifth month is Boys' Day. Gigantic carp-shaped paper or cloth windsocks float over towns and villages.

Carp (*Koi*) swim upstream during spawning season. They represent "courage" and "perseverance," and are also a symbol of both love and virility. In China, where they originated, legend has it that the carp that swam the entire length of the Yellow River against the current turned into dragons.

In Didier Decoin's novel *The Office of Gardens and Ponds*[43] a fisherman's widow undertakes a perilous journey through 12th century Japan to take baskets overflowing with ornamental carp to the Imperial Palace, just as her husband would have. Carp – red, white, yellow, black, and white with red and black spots – bring beauty and serenity to gardens.

On Boys' Day at the Murai's, models of samurai and heroes of the past would have been set out on display. It would be iris season, and irises would have been placed in the baths to chase away evil spirits. Mrs. Murai would have prepared two rice dishes, *chimaki* (steamed rice wrapped in bamboo leaves) and *Kashiwa mochi* (rice cakes stuffed with bean paste and wrapped in oak leaves).

In the snow a globefish
The left team wins with
A carp in June

– *Basho*

June 10 is "Punctuality Day," in memory of Emperor Tenchi (661-672) who had the temple bells ring out every hour of the day. Prior to that, time was indicated through reference to the sun: dawn, morning, mid-day, evening, and night. Emperor Tenchi introduced the first water clock (clepsydra), to measure time and divide it into equal parts, a system already in use in China. Day and night combined were divided into twelve units that varied with the seasons, with each unit corresponding to two hours in our system. The units were named after the animals of the zodiac: the hour of the Rabbit, the hour of the Ox, etc. The Japanese language is averse to precision. To define something is to bring it to a standstill and threaten its very existence. Life is a never-ending transformative process and that movement must not be arrested. The very notion of exactitude is offensive to the Japanese temperament. When making an appointment people say, "Around ten, but be on time!" If you give family or friends a specific time you limit their freedom and make them uncomfortable; the celebration will start in the evening, or early in the morning, or whenever everyone gets there. In 1920, in order to facilitate life at the work place, the government launched a national campaign to promote respect for time. On "Punctuality Day," citizens are asked to set their watches and avoid being vague.

At daybreak
A woman holds onto her man
With grace and tact

– *Basho*

With June comes the rain. In anticipation of mold season, houses are given a thorough cleaning and clothes are put away in tightly sealed trunks or closets. Once the rain has abated, doors open wide and everything is hung outside to dry in the sun and prevent germs from spreading.

Farmers welcome the rain, torrential though it often is, for it is beneficial to rice crops. The grains of rice that were sown at the beginning of May, exactly 88 days after *Setsubun* in early February, have sprouted by June and the seedlings are tall enough to be replanted in fields saturated with lukewarm water.

As promised, Kyoko sent me a picture of the rice paddy that was just a mud field when we saw it during our travels.

Intermittent rain
No need to worry
About rice seedlings

– *Basho*

On the other hand, people working in sericulture dread the rain season. Not far from Doctor Inasaka's clinic, on the site of what is now a mountain climbing museum, there used to be a cocoon farm. When Jiro Murai started out he studied silkworm rearing. Perhaps that is where his vocation came from. In all events, dampness is often fatal to silkworms, which are highly sensitive to abrupt changes in temperature. Sericulturists need to be extremely vigilant. They keep their warehouses heated to accommodate the valuable worms teeming on shelves covered with straw and mulberry leaves.

The Only Son is a 1936 film by Yasujiro Ozu. We see a posted sign at the entrance to the village announcing the spring sale of silkworms, and a procession of women in kimonos and conical hats approaching with boxes of these precious creatures carried on their backs.

June drizzle
The leg of the crane
Becomes shorter

– *Basho*

Irises and lotus flowers bloom in late June, when the great festival is held at the Atsuta Shinto shrine, in Nagoya, said to be the repository of the famous *Kusanagi-no-Tsurugi,* "Grass-Cutting Sword." It, along with the *Yata-no-Kagami* ("Mirror of Justice") and the *Yasakani-no-Magatama* ("Jewel of the Five Hundred Branch Tree"), are the Three Sacred Treasures of Japan.

As with a number of swords that are objects of worship in Japan, *Kusanagi-no-Tsurugi,* the Magical Sword, is believed to have divine powers. The Japanese were excellent metalworkers, and steel was all the more precious because to make it required all five elements: earth, metal, fire, water, and wood. In the Middle Ages, each European knight had his faithful sword, whereas in Japan it was the samurai warrior who was faithful to his sword, the blade of which represented purity. In Ueda Akinari's short story "Lust of the White Serpent" (in *Tales of Moonlight and Rain*), a fisherman's son gives a beautiful young woman a sword stolen from a monastery. Wherever he goes, he finds himself pursued by this young woman who has turned into a snake. He has to enlist the help of a high priest to rid the sword of the demon inhabiting it.

That thrust of the sword
Did I really dream it
Flea bites

– *Takarai Kikaku* (1661-1707)[44]

The seventh day of the seventh month is *Tanabata*, the Star Festival, which celebrates the reuniting of Vega and Altair. Vega was a weaver who crafted beautiful pieces of fabric for her father, the king of Heaven. One day, the shepherd Altair came to visit and the two of them fell in love. Vega began neglecting her loom. The wrathful father put an end to the romance, banishing them to opposite ends of the heavenly river, but allowed the two lovers to reunite once a year, on the seventh day of the seventh month. But to do so, Vega and Altair had to travel across the Milky Way, and the distance proved too great. As they bemoaned their fate, magpies formed a bridge between them with their wings. Vega, the weaver, became somewhat of a goddess of the arts and feminine crafts, of poetry, and of music. People pray to both of them for success in love.

Rainy Star Festival
The weaver and the shepherd cannot meet
Bliss of rain

– Basho

On July 15, as schools are about to close for the summer, *O-bon*, the Lantern Festival, or the Day of Souls, begins. The spirits of the dead come home for three days to visit their families. To help them find their way, people hang lanterns by the door. There was a time when people would hold feasts in cemeteries. Elaborate little boats, with lanterns hanging from their masts, would be loaded with food and set afloat on rivers or at sea, to carry the spirits of the dead back to the Beyond. There would be singing and dancing and fireworks illuminating the sky. In Hirokazu Kore-Eda's *Still Walking*, we see the Yokoyama family assemble to honor the memory of their first son, who died while saving a child from drowning.

It is a time for revisiting memories and words that went unspoken and that cloud relationships between parents and children.

Wake up wake up
Be my companion
Oh sleeping butterfly

– Basho

In mid-July, Tokyoites feel compelled to eat smoked eel. According to an ancient saying, whoever eats *unagi* on the day of the Ox during *doyo* (the hottest period of the year) will be spared all manner of illness for the rest of the summer. The eel is an odd fish with a way of life veiled in mystery. Eels spawn in open sea and it takes months for their young to reach the shore. Once there, they grow into fingerlings and begin swimming upstream. Eels are of high nutritional value, with vitamin A and

E, protein, calcium, and iron. Japan is the largest consumer of eels in the world and has been for a long time. I had eaten some as a child, and the memory of it was not at all pleasant, but Kyoko taught me to appreciate the taste.

Only the Japanese would ever think of having an eel for a pet and only a Japanese director would choose an eel for his main character. Shoshei Imamura's *The Eel*, winner of the Palme d'Or at the Cannes Film Festival in 1997, is a film that is at once tragic, burlesque, and poetic. "Why an eel?" the bonze asks Yamashita. "Because it listens to what I say and never utters an unnecessary word." Yamashita has been released on parole after serving eight years for the murder of his wife.

No longer a man
Not yet an eel
Rain in June.

– *Kaneko Tota* (1897)

Fall, Winter Celebrations and Traditions Magical 8

The Japanese love the number 8. In a Tokyo pet shop, I even found a toy in the shape of an 8 for my cat. The Japanese archipelago includes eight islands, says the *Kojiki*, and there are eight million kami in Shintoism, 8 signifying a countless multitude. The oriental scholar Jean Herbert said: "In the *Kojiki* alone, 8 appears fifty times and 80 eighteen times, whereas the presence of other numbers does not exceed half a dozen. [...] However, ancient texts suggest that 8 and its multiples are most often mentioned to convey the combined notion of perfection and completion."[45]

Note, too, that the mathematical symbol for infinity is a horizontal 8.

In Jin Shin Jyutsu, the eighth depth is the source of all sources out of which there emerges the universal energy that created the Sun in the seventh depth. Jiro Murai placed safety energy lock 8 on the lateral side of the knee. The number 8 facilitates reproductive functions and elimination. It also releases muscle tension, and is associated with rhythm, strength, and peace in the universe. Find your strength in your rhythm!

On the medial side of the knee, we find safety energy lock 1, called "the primal cause." Placing your hands on it helps move energy downward, establishing harmony from head to toe. *Ichi* - 1 or first - is the greatest number of all. It encompasses everything, connects heaven and Earth, spirit and body, the highest heights and the deepest depths. It is thought to be the number most likely to bring good fortune.

秋
Autumn

According to the Chinese calendar, fall begins on August 8. It is associated with the color white and with downward movement. It marks the beginning of the yin phase of the year.

Father and mother
Often in my thoughts
The pheasant's call

– *Basho*

Kyoko goes back to Kyoto every year in mid-August to celebrate *O-bon*. The morning of August 16, she sent me pictures of the Heian Jing shrine, of her family, and their extraordinary *O-bon* dinner. This Celebration of the Souls has its roots in an Indian Buddhist ceremony, Ullambana, and in legend: in a dream, a man sees his mother literally starving to death. He brings her a bowl of rice that immediately turns into a bowl of fire. The dream is interpreted by a bonze to mean that the mother has committed sins in her previous lives. Because only Buddha's benevolence can spare her these torments, the son performs ceremonial prayers to restore peace to her soul. In another dream, the mother thanks her son, reassuring him that she is now free. Introduced at the Imperial court in 657, the custom reached into the population as a whole in the 10th century.

Nagisa Oshima's *Empire of Passion* (1978) is set in a rural village in northern Japan in 1895. During the *O-bon* festival, a man's ghost returns to haunt his widow and the lover who murdered him.

The pine wind
Circling around the eaves –
Autumn deepens

– *Basho*

Autumn is the most beautiful season of all.

Wisps of mist drift over the landscape and settle deep into valleys, inspiring painters. Art galleries and museums organize major exhibits. It is the time of chrysanthemums and ambient melancholy, and the time of weddings and pilgrimages, too. But for farmers and fishermen, the dreaded typhoon season lingers on. On September 18, Kyoko wrote, "We've just had our eighteenth typhoon. Two people died and three are missing. Tokyo is suffering from sweltering heat following last night's upheaval." The 210th (*Nihyaku-toka*) and 220th (*Nihyaku-hatsuka*) days after the beginning of spring are especially feared. In North America, hurricanes are identified by common first names whereas in Japan they are given numbers, beginning at the start of the calendar year.

In Hirokazu Kore-Eda's film *After the Storm* a writer turned detective comes to visit his mother with his ex-wife, who is about to get remarried, and their son. The mother asks them to stay the night because a storm has broken the French window. The film's premise offers insight into the everyday life of a middle-class Japanese family as well as into the mutually inflicted wounds that undermine the serenity of relationships.

This autumn sunset
So like
The Land of Shadows

– *Basho*

September begins with the mournful remembrance of the Great Kanto Earthquake of 1923, which leveled the city of Tokyo, killing nearly sixty thousand people. In far more recent times, in March 2011, Japan suffered a threefold calamity: an earthquake followed by a tsunami that led to the Fukushima nuclear disaster in which 15,881 people died and 2,668 disappeared. One of the first things Kyoko told me when I came to live with her was, "The house is earthquake-proof, but if you feel it shaking, duck under a table. I never drain the bathwater at night, in case of fire. You never know." On television, the elderly are advised to carry a whistle at all times so they can signal their presence should their house collapse on them. On average, there is one major earthquake every three months. The archipelago as a whole undergoes about a thousand of them a year, or two or three a day. The Japanese all carry within them the memory of the chaos they sow and a deep sense of the impermanence of things. In his collection of short stories *After the Quake*,[46] Haruki Murakami explores the powerful tremors that devastate his characters from within.

Anniversary
Of the great earthquake
All my books all hold their breath

– *Nakamura Kusatao* (1901-1983)

September 9, the ninth day of the ninth month, is Chrysanthemum Festival (*Choyo*), called "Double Yang Festival" in China. Chrysanthemums were grown in China as early as the 15th century B.C.E. and were brought to Japan around the 8th century C.E. They are an essential element of Chinese pharmacopeia and are cited in the *Shen Nong Ben Cao Jing*, the oldest book on herbal medicine. Chrysanthemums are good for the liver, the eyes, high blood pressure, and headaches. They are also said to prolong life.

After the mums
There is nothing left
But the daikon

– *Basho*

In Japan, Chrysanthemum Day is known as the "Festival of Joy." The chrysanthemum is a sacred flower and serves as the emblem of the Imperial family. The Japanese Imperial seal, literally the "chrysanthemum seal," was adopted by the Emperor Go-Toba (1180-1239) and still appears on passports. The Order of the Chrysanthemum is the highest honor one can receive.

Every other September 11, the Ginger Festival opens in the Shiba district of Tokyo. In the past, people suffering from eye ailments would devote their lives to selling ginger, which is reputed to combat visual deficiencies. In the area around Sadaki Kato's clinic there are stores that sell sesame seeds exclusively. They have been present in Japan since 1500 B.C.E. and Hippocrates recommended the seeds for their exceptional nutritional value. Nearby, I also saw lingerie shops teeming with older people eager to dress in red. The color is reputed to increase energy levels and resolve bladder issues, and is generally considered a protection against evil spirits and illness. It is the dominant color in all shrines.

The Great Festival of the Hachiman Shrine in Kamakura takes place from September 14 to 17. The shrine was dedicated to the Minamoto clan kami and flourished at the end of the 12th century under Minamoto-no-Yoritomo military rule. The festival is known for its historical reconstructions, especially its mounted archery competition. Hachiman is associated with Emperor Ojin who, according to both the *Kojiki* and the *Nihonshoki*, was the fourth son of Emperor Chuai and his wife, Empress Jingu. He is the first Emperor of Japan recorded in history, those who preceded him being the stuff of legend. He was said to have lived a hundred years and to have reigned for more than forty. When his first temple, Osai-no-miya (*yawata*) was built, eight banners are said to have floated down from the heavens. Hachiman Daimyojin is also known as Yahata-no-kami, the "God of Eight Banners."

The night is endless
I think of
What will come in 10,000 years

– *Masaoka Shiki*[47]

The full moon in September is a benevolent divinity inspiring calm and gentleness. The moon greatly influences the way we divide time. The Chinese lunar calendar, *Inreki*, remained in use until 1873, when Japan adopted the Gregorian calendar. In the past, ceremonies honoring the moon found people simply gathering to watch it, poets reading their latest haiku, and everyone eating fruit, *O-dango* rice balls, and other delicacies. In the full circle of the moon, it was customary for children to see a rabbit grinding rice in a mortar.

On September 3, Kyoko sent me pictures of the moon playing hide and seek with the clouds, as well as one of offerings made to the moon, and another of a reproduction of *The Square Light of the Moon* on a piece of cloth. In traditional homes, the image of the moon shines through the translucent panes of sliding partitions, *shoji*.

Open the lock
Let the moon shine in
Floating Temple

– *Basho*

October 10, the tenth day of the tenth month, marks *Kakashi-Matsuri* or the Scarecrow Festival. To thank Inari, the rice kami – a munificent and extremely popular kami – scarecrows are gathered in farmyards and adorned with a new set of clothes. Offerings, food, and work tools are placed at their feet. People do kami dances, stamping their feet to imitate the spirits of the fields.

Kaneto Shindo's *The Naked Island* (1960) is an ode to nature and telluric forces, much along the lines of Robert J. Flaherty's *Man of Aran*. On a tiny island, a father, mother, and their two sons work relentlessly to cultivate an arid piece of land. Daily life revolves around their need for water: they scull out to sea, scoop out buckets of water, carry them on their backs, carefully negotiate the steep slopes… day in and day out, the same movements order their lives and the seasons.

Much like men
Scarecrows in the moonlight
So pitiful

– *Masaoka Shiki*[48]

October 22 is the Festival of the Ages or *Jidai Matsuri*. It was inaugurated in 1895 for the 1,100th anniversary of the founding of Kyoto, then called Heian-Kyo. It commemorates the transfer of the Imperial capital from Nara to Heian-Kyo in 794. A magnificent procession of people dressed in age-old costumes moves from the Imperial Palace to the Heian Jingu Shrine.

Even in Kyoto
When I hear the cuckoo
I long for Kyoto

– *Basho*

In Tokyo, fall marks the beginning of a new season of sumo tournaments.

Pilgrimage to the tombs
The youngest child
Carries the broom

– *Issa*[49]

At the fall equinox, the sun sets due west. On *Higan* day, people pray so that the souls of the departed may travel safely to the "other shore," to the Pure Land of Amida Buddha. In Tokyo, at the equinox, people go to dog and cat cemeteries and pray for their pets' souls. Naoko, Kyoko's sister, dedicated a small altar to her dog, Mio. In *A Cat, A Man, and Two Women* (1936),[50] Junichiro Tanizaki reflects on the superiority of an animal's love over romantic or conjugal love. In *Mélodie,* Akira Mizubayashi pays homage to his dog: "I have turned a cupboard into a shrine that in no way looks like a normal shrine. It is now the resting place of souls both unforgettable and unforgotten. That is where I put a little lacquered wooden box for tea with a tiny portion of my father's ashes that I removed from his urn before it was placed in the grave. Eighteen years ago now, when I prepared this little coffer, I was brave enough to taste the ground bones. Soon, I will do the same for Mélodie, whose urn I still keep close by, in the exact spot where she had her mattress. I'll get another lacquered box and put in a few spoonfuls of powdered bone and a piece of shoulder blade or rib. I'll spread the rest in the garden or somewhere else where it can return to the earth."[51]

冬
Winter

On the Chinese calendar, winter begins on November 8. Its color is black and its movement inward and introspective. It marks the height of the yin phase of the year.

Reading Week begins on November 3, and with it the celebration of culture. Sugawara-no-Michizane (845-903), also known as Tenmangu Kan Shojo and Tenjin, was a scholar, poet, and politician of the Heian period. He was later deified as Tenjin, the kami of Learning. He was also said to possess the gifts of a healer.

Every year at the time of the Nobel prize, fans of Haruki Murakami gather at the Rokuijigen café, formerly a jazz bar, in the Ogikubo district of Tokyo, not too far from where Kyoko lives. When the recipient is announced, a wave of disappointment sweeps through the crowd, after which life begins anew and the Harukists savor some of the unique culinary creations described by their author. That year, 2017, the Nobel Prize in Literature was awarded to the British writer of Japanese descent, Kazuo Ishiguro, whom I discovered in 1987 while writing a review of *An Artist in the Floating World* for a magazine. A Japanese painter struggles to find meaning in life in the aftermath of WWII.

One of the last festivals of the year is *Shichi-go-san*, literally "7-5-3," thus named because it celebrates all children who turned seven, five, and three the previous year. It is a rite of passage that dates back to the Heian period. In Japanese numerology odd numbers bring good fortune. Jiro would have put on his finest kimono and been taken to a shrine in the hopes of receiving the benevolent oversight of the gods. In ancient Japan 3 year-old girls had their hair tied and put up for the first time; at five, little boys received their first trousers (*hakama*); and at 7 little girls put on their first wide obi. Children savor *chitose ame* ("thousand-year-old candy"), thin long red and white candy sticks that symbolize growth and long life.

Bowing and laughing
From her chignon
Falls a pellet

– Natsume Soseki[52]

The holiday season ends on November 23 with *Kinro-Kansha-no Hi*, Labor Thanksgiving Day. Long ago, the Emperor would make an offering of the year's first rice to the kami. Today, people find joy thinking back on the work they accomplished during the year.

Cold too, the gums
Of the salted sea bream
At the fishmonger's

– Basho

On December 8, schools used to ritualize the needles little girls had broken during the year by sticking them into tofu. The tradition eventually came to include all the objects sacrificed to man's labors – sculptors' tools, pieces of cherry wood used to engrave seals, etc. – and were honored in temples.

Kintsugi is the art of mending broken objects with threads of gold. It is a way of elevating objects to a level of greater worth by including in them the mishaps that are part of their history. The repairs are not concealed. They are made conspicuous so as to allow objects to begin a new cycle of life. The sublimation of pain is an art which in psychology is a sign of resilience.

Impossible to thread
The needle
I gaze at the blue sky

– *Ozaki Hosai*[53]

On December 14, a solemn service is held at the Sengaku-ji temple in an old district of Tokyo in memory of the forty-seven samurai who, in 1703, in an act of total honor and loyalty, committed suicide after avenging the offense their master had suffered. *Rônin* means "samurai without a lord." The vengeance of the forty-seven *rônins* was more than two years in the planning, during which time they affected a life of debauchery and gambling. When they stormed Kira Yohinaka's mansion and cut off his head, the shogunate sentenced them to commit *seppuku*. *The 47 Ronins* is a national legend related by Osaragi Jiro in his thousand-page-long novel.

Before committing *seppuku*, a warrior would make a speech and, if possible, recite a farewell poem.

Now crossing the world here below
In the moss of Takamatsu
Leaving my reputation as a samurai

– *Sihimizu* (1582)[54]

Winter represents the end of life. It is a time to seek refuge beside benevolent spirits and deities, and to honor one's ancestors. During the Nara period (710-784), people were recognized for reaching 40, 50, 60, or 70 years of age. According to Confucius, a forty-year old man is sure of himself. In Japanese, 42 is associated with the idea of death. The number 77, or *kiju*, joins the ideas of pleasure and longevity, and the number 88, *beiju*, also called Rice Celebration, those of rice and longevity. During birthday celebrations, people eat red bean rice, *sekihan*, with sea bream, *tai*, which is synonymous with luck.

Like most everywhere in the world, wisdom is passed on in the form of proverbs, often not unlike those of our own culture:

Those who predict the future do not know theirs.
Good medicine tastes bitter.
People with the same illnesses easily get along.
If you speak about a person, his shadow will soon appear.
Water always takes the shape of the vase.
Even Buddha will be offended if provoked three times.

In the past, the winter solstice, *Toji*, was celebrated on December 22 or 23. Artists, poets, musicians, and calligraphers would go to the Imperial palace to present their work. The bath water was flavored with yuzu, a kind of bitter orange, good for colds in winter. Eating summer pumpkin that day was said to ward off illness the following summer.

The end of the year is gift-giving season, *O-seibo*. It is customary to give gifts to your in-laws, your bosses, the family doctor… and the convention can now be transacted online. Today, an *O-seibo* gift is supposed to be worth 5,000 yen. Previously, it was to have a value of 3,000 yen (about $25) but never 4,000, for it has to be an odd number; even numbers are divisible by two and thereby symbolize division and the end of relationships. The same holds for gifts given at weddings and funerals, where money is put in special envelopes tied with a ribbon that is never to be used again.

Omisoka is the last day of the year. People eat buckwheat noodles, *soba*, often without soup but occasionally with duck breast. Seated around an elegantly dressed table, people draw the animal of their astrological sign on their chopstick sleeve. It is a time to repay outstanding debts. Houses are thoroughly cleaned and the paper covering *shoji* screens is changed. Kyoko has told me that it is a festive time for the family. Children love to tear off the old paper and watch adults put new paper on.

Afterwards, they put on new clothes and vacate the house for the night, so that demons can withdraw and good spirits can come and settle in their place.

Buddhist temples chime midnight by striking a large bell one hundred and eight times, 108 being the number of disturbing thoughts a human can harbor.

Morning of the New Year
How glamorous I look
In this new kimono

– *Basho*

Jin Shin Jyutsu says: Evolution is the law of life, numbers are the law of the universe, and unity is the law of the creator.

Hakusan
Ginkgos and Silkworms
Vocation

Suddenly the sky cleared and there it was at last, Hakusan, brilliant in the sunlight. Covered with its eternal snows, it is one of the three sacred mountains of Japan, along with Mount Tate and Mount Fuji. We were strolling aimlessly down the riverbank. In a week or two, the cherry trees would be in blossom. I took Kyoko across the river to take a picture of a ginkgo tree that I found even more majestic than the one at Dr. Inasaka's house. The ginkgo is descended from the world's oldest family of trees and has survived the dinosaurs and Hiroshima. Here it stood guard over the entrance to a beautiful old home; it is even reputed to have saved it from fire. The house was home to the mountain climber and writer Kyuya Fukada (March 11, 1903 – March 21, 1971). We were just in time for the last tour. We took off our shoes and put on slippers. In his introduction to the man who wrote the well-known *One Hundred Mountains in Japan*,[55] our guide quoted him: "Like a protective deity, there is a mountain in the heart of every Japanese." I imagined Jiro Murai driving a piton into a mountain face, roped up with Kyuya Fukada, the Japanese Erri de Luca,[56] while the latter recited his haiku. Murai could have met him in Kaga City where he was born, or in Tokyo where he studied and started his life as a writer by founding a literary review.

My mountain, the one I gaze upon from my window at sunrise and at sunset, is the Grand Veymont (7,680 feet), the highest point of the Vercors Massif. From its summit you overlook Mont Aiguille, which is said to be the birthplace of mountaineering in 1492. Mount Haku (8,860 feet) is a volcano. Its first eruption dates back 400,000 years, and its last to 1659, not long before Basho traveled through the region (1689). Our guide left us to watch a short black and white film about Fukada and two of his friends, Takami Jun and Hori Tatsuo, both writers like himself. Fukada signed his haiku Kyusan, literally "nine mountains."

Just before the end of the tour, the guide opened the doors to a cocoon cabinet. The house had once been a silkworm farm. Kaga was a city of weavers, its damp climate lending itself to the trade. Threads do not easily break in the damp. Mr. Shinohara would later explain to us that whereas cocoons are fragile and do not do well in such a climate, the thread, once it has been pulled free, needs the damp. There were once six silkworm workshops on that street alone, and when Mr. Shinohara was a child about thirty of them in Kaga, whereas today only one remains.

And we were in it!

Here, as a child, Murai would have been rocked to sleep by the hum of the looms. He might have found his calling here – as the second son, he would have been allowed to choose not to be a doctor. We know for a fact that he studied silkworm rearing (*kaiko*).

It was a traditional occupation, if there ever was one. At the time, it was said that Japan had been producing the most beautiful silk in the world for more than a thousand years. It was the occupation of the future too. In 1910, Japan was the world's leading producer of silk.

And it was a scientific occupation as well. *The Bombyx Mori*, the mulberry bombyx, which originated in China, is not found in nature. It is selectively bred through a process called sericulture. In its caterpillar stage, the bombyx produces an abundant stream of saliva that solidifies into a single thread of raw silk, between 800 and 1500 yards long, with which the cocoon is built. In Alessandro Barrico's novel *Silk,* the protagonist, the silkworm merchant Hervé Joncour, embarks on a perilous journey to Japan in 1861, at a time when disease was ravaging French silkworm farms. As we follow Joncour on his various expeditions we come to realize how precious and fragile silkworms are. To be a skilled silkworm engineer requires specific abilities: the ability to observe, to be meticulous and rigorous, and to enjoy the role of caregiver. Silkworms have inspired modern biology since 1865 when Louis Pasteur and his team set up a lab on a silkworm farm and developed the process of "cell seeding" to combat pébrine.

蚕
Silkworms

Devising Jin Shin Jyutsu required a deep understanding of the workings of the human body. Jiro Murai was clearly a brilliant mind with the indomitable spirit of a researcher.

When we got back to Tokyo, we learned from Sadaki Kato that Jiro Murai had attended one of the elite schools of the capital. Could it have been the sericulture school founded by Takayamasha in 1884 and which closed in 1927, and where even French specialists from Lyon came to teach? The school was part of the Tomioka Silk Mill.

During our first trip to Japan, my husband and I visited with an old weaver living in a traditional house in Kyoto. He was almost a hundred years old, and magnificent in his brown kimono. He served us tea on his tatami and told us his life story. He had worked as an artisan weaver in the ready-to-wear industry for his entire career. On his retirement, he decided to pursue the same activity, but with an emphasis on art. He had woven a cloth depicting "The Tale of the Genji" in 11th century

Japan, much like the Bayeux tapestry recounts the history of 11th century France. He rolled out his creation in front of us, freshly completed after nearly thirty years of work. He wished to make a gift of it as a way of thanking France for the Jacquard machine that was perfected in Lyon in 1801.

It was teatime when we pushed open the door to a black house, a gemstone workshop where they also served food. Our hostess invited us to look at the gems on display, then showed us the studio. Her husband was cutting stones in an old dentist's office, using the dental equipment that had been left behind. We had been trying to meet Kaga's former mayor, whose father, a writer, had written several books on the region. Our hostess knew him very well. He lived nearby and now that he was retired frequently came by to learn about gem cutting. Kyoko immediately tried to talk to him on the phone, but he was in a foul mood that evening and wanted nothing to do with us. Our hostess then gave us the name of one of her friends, Riyuchi Shinohara, a historian who worked in the tourist office and who might be able to help. We arranged to meet with him the next day.

We had kept postponing our departure from Kaga, and that evening was no different. The room at the hotel was still available, and at the same reduced price.

The brazier was heated and the tourist office near the Daishoji station smelled from oil and rice. When he saw us, Mr. Shinohara stopped nibbling at his food and set down his bento. We had a very pleasant time with this historian and former school principal who took an avid interest in our quest. I was trying to get a sense of who Jiro Murai was before he became ill.

As a young man, Jiro might have participated in eating contests and might even have made money that way. At Yuko's restaurant, Kyoko engaged people at the bar. Were there still eating contests in the area? What were the trouser-busting foods these people stuffed themselves with? Rice balls filled with red bean paste (*daifuku*)? Buckwheat noodles? We were unable to get a satisfactory answer.

With a twinkle in his eye, Mr. Shinohara gave us to understand that our big eater was almost certainly a big saké drinker, too.

In her book *Introducing Jin Shin Jyutsu Is,* Mary Burmeister wrote that Jiro Murai "became terminally ill with an unknown illness. No one could be found to help him. His own family could do nothing but to watch him fade away."[57] In *The Touch of Healing, Energizing Body, Mind, and Spirit with the Art of Jin Shin Jyutsu,* Alice Burmeister and Tom Monte said, "A succession of doctors treated him, but his condition only worsened until he was pronounced incurable and given up for terminally ill."[58]

Pronounced terminally ill at twenty-six years of age… What doctors were making these diagnoses? Ranpo or Kampo?

In the work that Kyoko later translated for me, Haruki Kato wrote that Jiro's father and brother, both doctors, sent him to a professor of medicine at Tokyo University (unfortunately, no name is given). To no avail.

Jiro Murai must have been treated by Western, Ranpo doctors.

What was he suffering from?

Typhoid, like the physician Hakaru Hashimoto (1881-1934), the artist Gyoshu Hayami (1894-1935), or the great legal scholar Ume Kenjiro (1860-1910)?

A malignant tumor, like the writer Nakae Chomin, who, knowing his days were numbered, devoted the time he had left to write *A Year and a Half.*

Bone tuberculosis, like Masaoka Shiki, who wrote the sickbed diary, *A Drop of Ink*.

Gastric hemorrhaging, like Natsume Soseki, the famous author of *Recollections* (*Omoidasu koto nado*).

Syphilis, like Guy de Maupassant, the French writer whom Kyoko Watanabe presented a paper on at a conference at the University of Brest, in 2013.

Perhaps mental illness, Mr. Shinohara said. Was he suggesting alcoholism?

Drunken Angel (1948) is Akira Kurosawa's first "great" film (1948). Against a backdrop of total destitution, it portrays the antagonistic relationship between an alcoholic doctor and a gangster with tuberculosis who understand each other perfectly.

Emperor Meiji died in 1912, and was succeeded by his son, the crown prince, Emperor Taisho (1879-1926). Taisho was of fragile health. He suffered from the cerebral meningitis he contracted three weeks after he was born.

At the time, many illnesses were not diagnosed as precisely as they are today.

Meditation
Sacred Mountain
Revelation

In 1912, at age twenty-six, Jiro Murai apparently asked to be taken to a mountain cabin. At what time of year was this? Alice Burmeister and Tom Monte wrote that, "As a last request, he asked his family to carry him on a stretcher to their mountain cabin and to leave him there alone for seven days. He asked that they return for him on the eighth day."[59] Mary Burmeister similarly said, "He finally requested his family to carry him on a stretcher up to their mountain cabin. He wanted to be alone. He asked them to leave him in solitude for seven days and to return on the eighth day to see the outcome."[60]

Mr. Shinohara said that in the Kaga region families do not have mountain cabins. He rather thought that Jiro, the bad son, the dissolute rapscallion, might have contracted a disease thought to bring shame on the family and been banished as a result, which was common practice at the time. Even if a banished son or daughter were to make amends, they were never allowed to return home. That might explain why the details of Jiro Murai's life are so scarce. (I immediately seized upon this hypothesis).

Back in Tokyo, Kyoko read in Haruki Kato's book that when Jiro Murai realized he was terminally ill he said, "I want to be taken to the mountains and be left there to starve to death. I don't want anyone to know." The request left his relatives dumbfounded, but he was adamant and they did as he asked. He was living in Tokyo then, with his pregnant wife. It is thought he left her a letter giving her back her freedom. Was the letter enough to annul the marriage? In Hayao Miyazaki's animated film *The Wind Rises*, two witnesses and three cups of saké are enough to make Jiro Horikoshi and Noaka's union official. My friends the Mizubayashis say that making a marriage or a divorce official is remarkably easy. One of their friends actually found out she was divorced well after the fact. When I expressed surprise that Jiro Murai would divorce his pregnant wife, Sadaki Kato explained that in those days it was more difficult for a widow to start a new life than a divorcee. Did Jiro Murai give his wife back her freedom out of pure generosity? After his recovery, he did not return to his family. His son died very young.

There is no indication of a family mountain cabin like the ones found in the French Alps. Mr. Shinohara thought that Jiro might rather have sought refuge in a counterfeiter's cave, like those near the top of the hill on the Road to the Seven Temples, or in a *dokoutsu*, a meditation cave dug into the mountainside for the practice of *zazen*. *Zazen*, literally "seated meditation," is a form of meditation intended to lead us to enlightenment (*satori*). The practice and the awakening are likened to the palm and the back of one's hand. Simply sitting still, in silence, creates a space in which one can be in harmony with Buddha's illumination. A Buddhist friend of mine explained that these meditation caves were rudimentary shelters. Some were made of wood, which might explain why they were translated as "cabins." Hermits would barricade themselves in with enough food to last as much as six months. While in Tibet, Jérémy heard the story of a terminally ill man who withdrew to a *dokoutsu* to purify his soul through prayer and meditation before dying. But the more he became enlightened, the more he regretted not having enjoyed the level of consciousness he had achieved while he still had his life to live. Time passed until finally one day, feeling himself healed, he broke down the door and returned to the world.

Haruki Kato said that once left alone Jiro Murai practiced *zazen*. "He thought that rather than just idly wait for death to come he would be better off meditating and doing the mudras, which he knew, *even though he had never actually studied them.*"

We left Mr. Shinohara and headed for the Road to the Seven Temples. A plaque informed us that Basho himself had walked that path. The first four temples were Buddhist, the fifth, Shinto. The Japanese are often both Shintoists and Buddhists. Whereas Shintoism involves honoring kami at festivals and pilgrimages, Buddhism is based on a complex body of doctrines. Over the centuries, the philosophies and ritual practices have become so intertwined that it is often difficult to say which tradition they belong to. Zen Buddhism, which originated in China, came to Japan in a series of waves between the 8th and the 13th centuries. It deeply influenced the samurai. Zen philosophy promotes being in the moment, the here and now, with neither hope nor fear.

Before leaving Ishikawa prefecture, we stopped in Kanazawa where Kyoko wished to visit the house of Daisetz Teitaro Suzuki (1870-1966), the Buddhist philosophy professor, Zen scholar, and historian who introduced Zen Buddhism to the West. He was well read by European philosophers like Martin Heidegger and Karl Jaspers, and hailed by people like the psychoanalyst Carl Jung: "Suzuki's writings on Zen Buddhism are among the best there are."[61]

Mikao Usui (1865-1926), who founded *reiki* – another form of Japanese alternative hands-on therapy – was born into a Buddhist family of the Tendai school that teaches a form of meditation based on mudras and mandalas. In 1922, the monk went on a twenty-one-day retreat on Mount Kurama to meditate and fast. Legend has it that the teachings of *reiki* came to him in a moment of enlightenment (*satori*) during those twenty-one days.

Morei Ueshiba (1883-1969) is the founder of aikido, a martial art with a strong spiritual component. He was a disciple of the Shinto sect of Omoto-kyo and dedicated much of his life to the study of *Kotodama,* a basic concept of Shintoism. The Omoto-kyo religion came into being with Nao Deguchi (1837-1918), an illiterate peasant endowed with shamanic powers. At age fifty, she fell into a trance that lasted for weeks. When she emerged, she began prophesying the misfortunes that were to mark the 20th century through a form of automatic writing in phonetic script (*hiragana*), and called for more humanity in the world through renewed spirituality. In 1892, she created a new religion based on the worship of the folk deity Ushitora-no-konjin ("Big Origin" or "Original Root"), who dates back even further than Amaterasu. The kami of Omoto (literally "great origin") is Ameno minaka Nushi, the supreme deity of Shintoism.

Having recovered from his illness, Jiro Murai began studying Shingon Buddhism, an esoteric Japanese school of Buddhism founded in the 9th century. Its principle is encapsulated in the phrase "*Nyojitsu chijishin*": Truth is about knowing one's own mind, as it really is.

霊峰
Sacred Mountain

The Ballad of Narayama

"Beyond mountain after mountain, in the distant reaches of the Shinano region, lies a forgotten valley with a meandering river so narrow it looks like a ribbon, the slender Itogawa. On its banks, the cicadas wax melancholic, singing the tale of a village from time immemorial now lost..." So sings the messenger in Keisuke Kinoshita's *The Ballad of Narayama* (Palme d'or in Cannes in 1983). The film recounts the legend of Obasute. The seventy-year old Orin asks her son Tatsuhei to carry her up Mount Nara on his back, as tradition dictates, so that she can die there in peace. He is reluctant to accede to her wishes and complies only after she smashes her teeth. One evening, the elders come by to offer counsel and prepare him for the journey. They kneel with their hands in their laps and articulate the rules he must obey. After each commandment, they pass around a bowl of broth and drink from it with a ladle. There are five men and a woman. Only three of them speak.

The oldest speaks first, "When you set out on your journey, make sure no one sees you."

The second one says, "On your way down from the mountain, never look back."

And the third one, "As for the path you will take, circle around behind the mountain. When you come to a holly tree, go around the next mountain. Climb up the third mountain until you reach a pond. Walk around it and head up the stone steps of a fourth one. When you reach the top, Messire Narayama will be on other side of the valley. Continue walking, with the valley on your right and the next mountain on your left. It is two and a half leagues around the valley, and there is a trail with seven bends in it in a place called the Seven Valleys. Once the Seven Valleys are behind you, you will be on the way to Narayama. In Narayama, there is a path, yet there is no path. Climb up among the oak trees, higher and higher… and there, god awaits you."62

The film was adapted from a novel by Shichirô Fukazawa (1914-1987), published in 1956.

Kato believed that when Jiro Murai was on the mountain he fasted, meditated, and practiced finger positions. He lost consciousness several times and his body temperature plummeted. On the sixth day, he was freezing cold and thought he would die. On the seventh, a burning sensation coursed through his body. When the intense heat finally receded he was overcome with an immense calmness and a vast inner peace. It was a struggle for him to get to his feet, but he eventually did. He tried to walk, and saw that he could. To his family's amazement, he said that he would walk down the mountain by himself. It had dawned on him that there might be a connection between the mudras and fasting. Although he had barely recovered, he began fasting and meditating anew and relived the same experience. He concluded that fasting while doing the mudras stimulated circulation in the body. He immediately began reading texts on mudras.

Mudra is a Sanskrit word meaning "seal," but the first part, *mud*, means "joy" and the second, *ra*, "to trigger." The mudras are an intrinsic part of Vedic culture and their origin dates back to the most ancient times (India, 3500 B.C.E.). In India they are regarded as the source of all knowledge. The teachings of the Vedas are accompanied by the practice of mudras, also called "sacred gestures," "mystic gestures," and even "magic gestures."

Mudras have spread throughout the world through dance, art, and sculpture as well as through Hindu and Buddhist spiritual practices and worship, meditation and yoga.

There are energetic pathways in our subtle body that govern both our physiology and our psychology. These channels mostly converge towards or emanate from the surface of our hands and feet. Our fingers are related to the five elements. By "working" with our fingers we can improve our physical condition, moderate our emotions, increase our concentration, and be in harmony with the universe.

Jiro Murai meditated for seven days and on the eighth he felt his health had improved. In astrology, the number 7 is used to delineate the different periods of one's destiny. Periods of seven days also mark the different phases in the progression of an illness. Seven (7) is the principle of evolution. Eight (8) is the double matrix; it signifies the shape of our astral body, and the state of nirvana and holiness.

Haruki Kato said that Jiro Murai fasted twelve times, each time for three weeks. He might also have practiced waterfall meditation.

Deep in the mountains of Japan, ascetics, hermits, and lay devotees (*upsaka*) have been engaging in this strangest of practices for thousands of years: meditating under ice-cold waterfalls (*takigyo*). The Buddhist priest and martial arts expert Sylvain Guintard-Kuban said that "Acts of asceticism beneath waterfalls generate the energy needed to promote healing.... That is why shamanic healers in Japan have made *takigyo* their ultimate ascetic practice."[63] Kyoko has seen stories about it on the news, for it is still practiced today.

Once he had these experiences, Jiro Murai began to sense clearly a fluid-like movement in his body. He then sketched out its pathways.

印相
Mudra

With Jin Shin Jyutsu, our life is in our hands.

Jiro Murai believed that simply joining our hands together unites body and spirit, that it connects our spiritual and physical beings, and solar and lunar energies. Simply bringing our hands together at the level of the heart, the heart chakra, engenders love and peacefulness, this mudra being both a request and an expression of gratitude. All mudras send energy throughout the body and give us the ability to deal with physical, mental, and emotional problems. In studying the similarity between hands and feet Jiro Murai discovered that they were energetically connected. He saw similarities between the three phalanges of the hand and those of the foot, as well as between the palm of the hand and the sole of the foot, and he uncovered a connection between opposing fingers and toes: the thumb and the little toe, the index and the second toe, and so on. Jin Shin Jyutsu teaches us that our ten fingers can regulate 14,400 bodily functions.

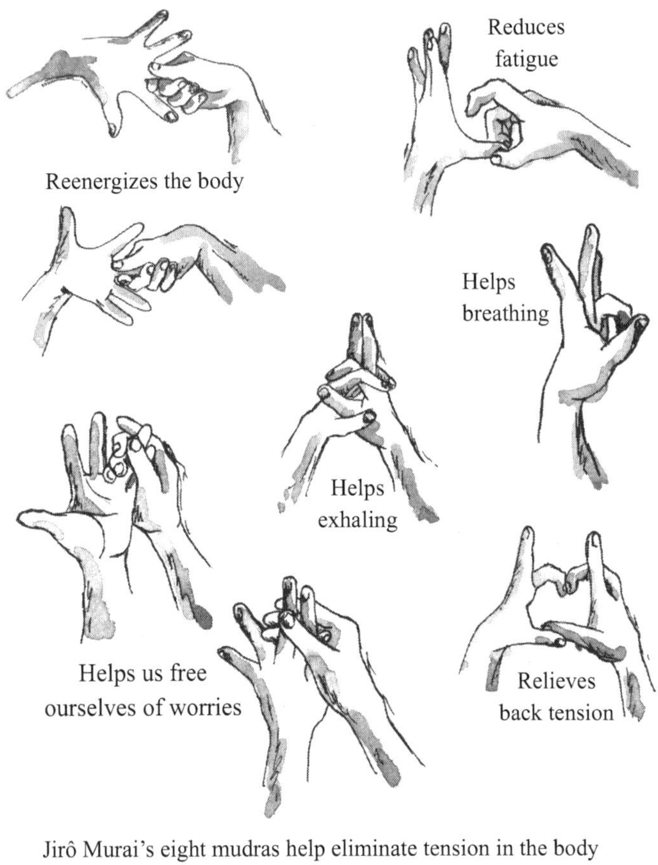
Reenergizes the body
Reduces fatigue
Helps breathing
Helps exhaling
Helps us free ourselves of worries
Relieves back tension

Jirô Murai's eight mudras help eliminate tension in the body
(in: Haruki Kato, note 33)

Samurai
Body and Soul
Harmony

The wind had picked up. We were strolling along the shore. Far away, beyond Korea, lay China. Before the Meiji era, Japan looked toward China alone, having closed its doors to the West. In Jiro Murai's day, ships loaded with rice would set sail towards Hokkaido and come back with holds full of herring and seaweed. This would be our last evening bath, our last dinner at Yuko's. The next time I come, I'll have my personal set of chopsticks and a flask of saké waiting for me under the counter. Yuko, who has three children, wanted to know how many I had. Her sister couldn't have any either. Had Yuko been younger, she would have given her sister one of hers. Luckily, her sister was happy in her marriage. She asked me if I was in mine. Thanks to Kyoko, we had no trouble communicating. Was it because we did not speak the same language that she felt comfortable asking me these things? This is exactly what I love about traveling: the encounters you have. On the surface, Yuko and I were worlds apart, yet the affinity ran deep; we were clearly sister souls. When it was time to leave, I wanted to take her in my arms. We bowed deeply instead.

Shortly before that moving moment of intimacy, we had spoken with a couple of regulars who were lacquer manufacturers. Lacquer is the natural sap of the lacquer tree. *Urushi* is a type of lacquer that dates back to the Jomon period (1,400-300 B.C.E.), when most of Japan's inhabitants were hunter-gatherers. Objects in *urushi* from Kaga became famous when, during the Edo period, Maeda Toshitsune, the third feudal chieftain of the Kaga domain, brought artisans from all over Japan to his court. *Urushi* was applied to wood, paper, and clothing as a protective coating. Even samurai armor was covered with it. In Kaga, house pillars and living room walls were traditionally lacquered in red, creating a stunning effect, as is the case at the former inn dedicated to the poet Basho. Our lacquer merchants are from Osaka, "a little like Southern Europeans," Kyoko whispered to explain their exuberance. They had never been to France, but they knew all the films of the Nouvelle Vague inside and out.

After a few cups of saké, "Mrs. Urushi" started singing *L'Eau Vive,* which she remembered from her French class, and I joined in.

The following day, we were to leave this region that would forever remain in our hearts. Since then, Kyoko and I have never been together without bringing up our trip here. We went to the library to say goodbye to Mrs. Shimizu. She had a bag full of bookmarks for us, little paper dolls crafted by her ninety-three-year-old mother. I inserted them in each of the eighty works I consulted in writing this book. The following day, we paid a parting visit to Alexandre Leroi, at the Tourist Office near the train station. He later wrote to me, "It was a pleasure to meet you. My colleagues are absolutely fascinated by your project and let me tell you, their search engines are going full blast on Jiro Murai. We'll keep you posted."

Did Jiro Murai even live in Kaga? Maybe Kaga is just the place the Murai family originally came from. Surely there was some way to gain access to Jiro Murai's *koseki,* but how? Kyoko, who taught in the Law Department at Meiji University, promised to look into it. On November 28, 2017, she wrote, "Do you remember what I told you about the *honseki* showing family roots? It turns out it is not that simple. A colleague of mine who is a legal expert said that you don't need to have family in a place to choose it for your *honseki*. Jiro Murai's *koseki* could be in Kaga, Tokyo, Kanagawa, or any other city in Japan!" Several months later, Kyoko showed me her *koseki,* which she had obtained from

Kyoto's City Hall, where her father was born and where the Watanabes are originally from. Kyoko herself was born in Osaka. It was a simple sheet of paper with a few horizontal lines of kanji. It included her father's name and her mother's married name, but there was no mention of her mother's maiden name nor of her older sister or of the latter's date of birth. Kyoko was simply listed as the second daughter, followed by her date of birth, the date it was recorded, and the name of the person who made the declaration of birth. Her father had gone to the Registry Office ten days after she was born, on June 28, and the information was officially recorded at City Hall on July 8. Had Watanabe-san made a point of having his daughter come into the world under the sign of the number 8?

The writer Akira Mizubayashi reminded me that there were no city halls in Jiro Murai's day; births were recorded in temples. His own father was sure of neither his birthdate nor his name, the spelling of which could have been inadvertently altered with a simple slip from one kanji to another. Before the Meiji era, every Japanese person had to belong to a Buddhist temple. The system had been put in place to keep track of Christians, then an oppressed people, and population movement. The bombings during World War II destroyed many official records and made it difficult to establish identities. The modern form of the *koseki* appeared in 1947, Akira said, while drawing a house in the air with his finger, a charming Japanese habit that often accompanies words that, as pronounced, can have several meanings. The modern *koseki* is limited to the nuclear family, that is, parents and their unmarried children. Akira Mizubayashi told me that Japanese law had not recognized his marriage with a French woman, Michèle, in the 1980s, and that he had remained on his parents' *koseki* until their daughter, Julia, was born.

The following day, we stopped in Kanazawa, an hour north of Kaga. It had been the fiefdom of the Maeda clan, one of Japan's most powerful families of samurai that had ruled Ishikawa Prefecture from 1583 to 1868. I would use the time to look into the *Bushido,* "the Way of Warriors," the samurai code of honor.

侍
Samurai

The *Way of Warriors* was the product of a long ethical evolution dating back to the 8th century. Originally, the samurai were highborn warriors serving feudal lords. Their status was hereditary; only a samurai's son could become one. Towards the end of the 16th century, when Akira Kurosawa's *Seven Samurai* takes place, Japan was ravaged by civil war. Lords began recruiting samurai from inferior castes. The samurai was schooled to defeat every enemy he faced, even if it meant giving his own life doing it. In 1585, the Jesuit Luis Frois wrote, "In our country, it is a sin to kill yourself, but when a Japanese warrior can take no more, he disembowels himself in what is considered an act of great bravery."[64] Clint Eastwood's *Letters from Iwo Jima* shows the influence of the samurai on Japanese soldiers during World War II. They choose to commit suicide rather than surrender to the enemy.

Today, the code of the samurai essentially focuses on the notions of honor and loyalty, and is taught in judo, karate, and kendo. The three pillars of the *Bushido* are *gishi* (rectitude), *giri* (duty), and *nin* (benevolence).

The following precepts, taken from the oath of the samurai, bring to mind Murai Sensei:

I have neither father nor mother; the heavens and the earth are my parents.

I possess no magical power; I have made my personality my magical power.

I have neither life nor death; my life and death are one.

I have no armor; I have made benevolence my armor.

I have no castle; I have made my unwavering mind my castle.

I have no sword; I have made my non-being my sword.

神
Kami

Shinto philosophy sees a soul in everything that exists in the universe. Kami, which translates as "deity," also means "breath," the essence of all forms of life. One has only to walk through Kenroku-en, the gardens in Kanazawa built by the Maeda clan between 1620 and 1840, to feel oneself filled with reverence before the gracefully gnarled bough of an ancient tree, or a torii opening onto a sacred space, or a team of gardeners in blue overalls and pointed hats hurrying over and squatting to brush away pine needles. In the temple here, on a sun-drenched afternoon, I placed a wooden ex-voto up above hundreds of others to ask Jiro Murai for help and inspiration.

Founded in 1583, Kanazawa, "marshes of gold," is the city of ancestral Japanese artisanry: ceramics, lacquerware, silk kimonos, Japanese paper… "Just looking at the texture of Chinese or Japanese paper brings a feeling of gentle warmth that soothes our hearts," Junichiro Tanizaki wrote in *In Praise of Shadows*. The "breath of life" flows through the master artisan's hands. The concentration, precision, and purity of his movements are the signs of its unspoken presence in what is and what has been crafted. Much like tea ceremonies, martial arts, and Noh theater, *washi* (paper making), *urushi* (lacquerware making), *ikebana*, and calligraphy are national treasures, veritable beings that are revered as such.

After a magnificent summer, winter suddenly descended upon the Vercors mountains. Summer vacation was drawing to a close. It was time to clean the house. My husband let me know he would be out in the barn, practicing archery. Daniel had taken to archery intuitively, at a fairground, when he was nine years old. Much to his surprise, he found that he *knew* how to shoot an arrow even though he had never used a bow before. He remembered the moment as a state of grace. He picked up archery again at age fifty, when we bought the house in the Vercors region. It is the only part of his life in which he feels bound by an inviolable rule. Only when he feels at one with the movement does he close his eyes and shoot.

There is an ancient saying in the art of archery (*kyudo*), "one shot, one life!" that captures this notion of the absolute that is supposed to inhabit our every action. Awa Sensei, the great master of *kyudo*, used to say, "If you want to live in harmony with heaven and Earth, which is the way of archery, don't try to reach the goal. Take no pleasure in the goal itself; follow the path to the union of body and soul ... *Kyudo* is a test of the self that is manifest in the relation between the target and the self."[65] Japanese masters are able to shoot their arrows in the dark or while riding a galloping horse, and hit the bull's eye, which, their teachings hold, is of secondary importance.

In Jin Shin Jyutsu, the practitioner's hands are guided by the "breath of life," which gives the practitioner's touch its soul. To develop this sensitivity without drawing on mental processes requires practicing accuracy and benevolence, as well as the will to generate harmony, which is a way of being devoid of will.

Mary Burmeister said, "... practice the art of Jin Shin Jyutsu with a pure mind in order to be the art itself."[66]

Sweet Bean
Master and Student
A Gift

Back in Tokyo, we had an appointment with Inaba Sensei at Regendo, a restaurant in the Ogikubo district known for its traditional Japanese cuisine. We had signed up for a cooking lesson to learn how to make fish stock. *Katshuobushi* is the Japanese name for skipjack tuna that is dried, fermented, and smoked. It is a basic ingredient in many soups, among them miso soup. We covered our hair with a cloth and put on aprons. Kyoko's apron was a kimono with puffed sleeves reminiscent of those you see in films. There were two other students there, a man and a woman. We bowed to each other. The chef was a totally bald and rather exuberant fellow. He was flattered to hear that I had come all the way from Paris for his class. Of Europe, he mostly knew London, where he had been invited to teach. He laid out his utensils. My eyes immediately lit upon a wooden implement that looked like a wood plane or a pencil box and that was used to shave *katsuo*, skipjack. Because shavings go bad quickly, it is best to shave them off as needed. In the past, it was imperative for young women to know how to shave *katsuo*, and brides were expected to bring their shaving boxes with them when they got married. Shaving boxes, which should never be washed, cost about 30,000 yen today. In Yasujiro Ozu's *Tokyo Chorus*, a mother kneels to shave *katsuo*. Inaba Sensei taught me the proper way to do it: you have to lean over the far end of the box, focus, hold your breath, grasp the *katsuo* tightly, and shave vigorously to obtain thinner or thicker shavings, as desired.

Skipjack is fished up and down the coast of Japan from spring to fall. As soon as they are caught they are boiled, after which they are skinned and deboned. Then they are sun-dried for 6 months until they become as hard as wood. The tradition dates back fifteen hundred years, and the recipe is found in the *Kojiki*.

The *katsuo* industry is made up of family businesses, and Inaba has been with the same family for thirty-five years. Of the various ways of catching shipjack, fishing with a rod and reel is best. Only the father is allowed to fillet fish and each fish cutter gives them his own signature shape. Nothing is wasted in the katsuo; the bones are sent to capsule manufacturers.

The teacher began to read his lesson, which gave rise to murmurs of approval. He mentioned that *katsuo* was not exported to Europe. Shortly after I got back to Paris, I went to visit my mother in Brittany. *Ouest-France*, a regional newspaper, was lying on the living-room table. An article caught my eye. "From Japan to Brittany… A Japanese manufacturer, Makurazaki, has recently opened a dried skipjack factory in Concarneau and plans to sell shavings in Europe of the same high quality as those sold in Japan." I promised myself I would have a look.

In French cooking, we have four essential tastes: sweet, salty, sour, and bitter. For the Japanese, there is a fifth one called *umami*, which literally means "savory." All of us have taste buds that specifically recognize the *umami* taste. At the beginning of the 20th century, a Japanese professor, Kikunae Ikeda, identified glutamate as the source of this taste. More recently, researchers have shown that glutamate is present in breast milk. It is also found in green tea, soy sauce, ripe tomatoes, and other foods such as *kombu* (dried seaweed), which is a staple of Japanese cuisine. To make *dashi* (fish stock) you need *kombu, katsuobushi* shavings, and shiitake mushrooms. In 1585, Luis Frois had already noted, "We don't have soup with our every meal, but the Japanese will not sit down to eat without a bowl of broth."[67]

Sweet Bean
Naomi Kawase's film (2015), based on Durian Sukegawa's novel *Sweet Bean Paste* (2013).
"You have to welcome them," Tokue says. "They took the trouble to come here." The old woman is talking about red beans. She has managed to get hired in a *dorayaki* shop to prepare red bean paste. "To start cooking them right away," she adds, "would be a lack of respect. They need time to get acquainted with the sugar. It is like an arranged marriage…"[68]

Leprosy had deformed Tokue's fingers and she had lived her entire life as an outcast, victim of the Leprosy Prevention Laws that were finally repealed in 1996. In the letter she wrote to Sentaro, the shopkeeper, who was the age the son she never had would have been, she said, "When I prepare *an*, the paste, I listen carefully to what the beans are saying. I try and imagine what they have gone through, the rainy days and the sunny ones. They made it all the way to us, carried by the wind. I listen to the tale of their journey. We truly need to listen to them. Everything that exists in this world has its own language. I am sure of it. The palest sunbeam, the faintest breeze… everything deserves to be listened to. "

Tokue would die of pneumonia and Sentaro would inherit her utensils. Tokue's final posthumous message was, "That day, the full moon whispered in my ear, 'I wanted you to look at me, that is why I am shining'."

先生
Teacher, Sensei

In his book on Jin Shin Jyutsu, Haruki Kato refers to Jiro Murai as *Sensei*. In classical Chinese, where the word comes from, it literally means a "person born before another." In Japan, the title

Sensei refers to "a person born before another and who possesses knowledge and experience in a particular field or of a particular skill." Today it is used in addressing a professor, doctor, or renowned artist, and is commonly applied to both sexes; Kyoko is called *Sensei*.

Haruki Kato became Jiro Murai's disciple during the twenty-eighth year of the reign of Emperor Showa, in 1953. Murai Sensei had started teaching a few years earlier, at the end of World War II, when Japan was rapidly becoming Americanized and its traditional cultural heritage had fallen into disfavor.

Haruki Kato spoke of his fervent admiration for Murai Sensei and his art. He had just turned twenty-five and was much younger than the other students. The Master's reputation had spread exclusively by word of mouth and barely went beyond the limited circle of initiates. Very few of the students truly intended to disseminate the teachings of Jin Shin Jyutsu. They were mainly there for the treatments. The medical profession had become tightly regimented under Emperor Meiji's rule. No one could open a practice without a university degree. One day, Haruki Kato told Murai Sensei, "I want to specialize in this." To which Jiro Murai Sensei replied, "If that is what you want, you will receive special training. However, you are not to study any other form of treatment until I say so. If you divert your attention elsewhere before you master the basics of Jin Shin Jyutsu you will mix things up and experience chaos."[69] Haruki Kato studied exclusively with Jiro Murai for three years, at the end of which Jiro Murai said, "Now go to acupuncture school and get a degree." While in school, Sensei taught him how to read acupuncture charts from the perspective of Jin Shin Jyutsu. Haruki Kato continued studying with him well after he had finished his course of study.

One day Jiro Murai told him, "I think my days are coming to an end. My pulses tell me that I have just two years left. You'll have to learn fast." Haruki quickly sorted out what he had learned and sought clarification for whatever he had not yet fully grasped. Sensei died two years later, in 1960, as he had predicted.

After his death, Haruki Kato encountered considerable resistance when he tried to use the name Jin Shin Jyutsu, which was often misinterpreted and associated with an esoteric sect. He named his clinic Jin Shin Do (House of the Virtues of the Body). Only after his book was published did he return to the name Jin Shin Jyutsu (Art of the Creator through man of knowing and compassion), out of loyalty to Jiro Murai. Jiro Murai believed that the art of Jin Shin Jyutsu is an innate part of man and was likely the starting point for acupuncture. After his teacher's death, Haruki Kato never stopped broadening his knowledge of Kampo medicine, first through the teachings of a certain Nishizawa, a nutrition expert, and then those of Kamei Susumu, who specialized in body movement and balance. He wrote his book not only to present Jin Shin Jyutsu to the world, but also to analyze the principles these different healing systems held in common. He taught at a college of acupuncture and at the Institute of Body Balance in Tokyo. When he started offering classes on Jin Shin Jyutsu to licensed therapists, his students all reacted positively. They saw the value of this art that could be applied effortlessly to people who were so seriously ill that they did not tolerate other therapies, such as acupuncture or shiatsu. Haruki Kato also trained his wife, and their son, Sadaki Kato, who has continued the practice.

In 1953, Mary Iino, who was to become the embodiment of Jin Shin Jyutsu in the West, teaching it, developing it, and making it widely known, went back to the United States to marry Gilbert Burmeister. She and her fiancé had met in the diplomatic corps. She was responding to the call of family life, but the decision to leave Japan was nonetheless a wrenching one. "To get married and create a family is a very important experience.

You'll be a richer person for it,"[70] Jiro Murai told her by way of encouragement. (He himself had separated from his wife in 1912. Nothing is known of his private life after that). She was thirty-five years old. She had come to Japan with General MacArthur's occupation forces and, still a young woman, participated in the creation of the first English language school. Her father, Uhachi Iino, a California businessman, had been interned in a detention center in 1941, after Pearl Harbor, along with thousands of other Japanese-Americans. There he learned about shiatsu from a fellow detainee and quite naturally shared his experience with his daughter. Before leaving Tokyo, Mary introduced him to Jiro Murai and the two men quickly became friends. Sensei was moved to hear that Mary spoke so highly of him and of Jin Shin Jyutsu. For nearly a year, Mr. Iino attended the same classes as Haruki Kato.

Jiro and Mary's father both had a deep knowledge of the Bible and enjoyed trading verses. Back in the United States, Mary's father died shortly after Murai Sensei. I have since come upon these words on page 2 of Mary's Text 2, just below the title "Physio-Philosophy (Nature-Effortless Reality): "In memory of Master Jiro Murai and my father."

In a filmed interview, Mary said that after meeting Jiro Murai she fell ill and was hospitalized, and that he came there to treat her. It is unclear what her illness was, but her condition appears to have been serious. Murai Sensei is supposed to have said, "What have you done to your precious body? This body needs to be looked after with care, attention, and common sense." He treated her for several weeks. The fourth week he said, "You will be up and about tomorrow." After which Mary became one of his most devoted students.

Mary studied with Jiro Murai for six years while performing her language-teaching duties. She continuously corresponded with him until his death. Like any life-changing encounter, theirs had something magical to it.

On the day they met, in 1946 or 1947 – I imagine it to have taken place in the spring, for I am of a belief that all important encounters take place in the spring – Murai has come unannounced to a house where Mary is scheduled to give an English lesson. She is standing outside, about to ring the doorbell. Inside the house, just as in Yasujiro Ozu's masterpiece *Tokyo Story* (1953), life has been thrown into turmoil. Everyone is bowing, the children have set aside their toys, the grandfather who was dozing on the tatami has been startled awake, and the woman of the house has interrupted her chores to put on the kettle.

Why has Murai Sensei come?

To listen to his patient's pulses? To confirm an intuition? For a treatment? They unfold the futon.

The doorbell rings.

Mary has closed the sliding door behind her, taken off her high-heeled shoes, and is about to step onto the tatami when her student greets her with his eyes aglow. "Murai Sensei is here," he whispers. "No one was expecting him. He never comes unannounced." There is nothing for her to do but turn around and leave. She'll come back another time. She begins to put her shoes back on.

With Sensei's curiosity aroused, he steps forward a little and looks at her through the translucent partition. Their eyes meet in the light of the *tokonoma*. Mary bows. Sensei bows. Mary bows again; both of them bow. Bowing once more, Sensei invites her to stay. Mary bows twice.

He is wearing a kimono and she, a narrow skirt and a white blouse. She kneels on a cushion. Tea is served on a lacquered table. She holds her little bowl in her hands. Jiro Murai is intrigued by this young American interpreter with whom he can communicate. Mary is interested in everything she is discovering in this, the land of her ancestors. She witnesses her first healing session and is profoundly moved. And yet, all Jiro Murai did was place his hands on his patient's body.

As they are about to say goodbye, without knowing anything about her, Jiro Murai bows and asks her if she would like to study with him and take a "gift" from Japan to America. Without knowing what he is actually talking about, she bows and replies, "Yes, Sensei."

Had Murai Sensei, who frequently came to that house, heard about the young woman's teaching skills? Had Mary, who often went there, heard about Jiro Murai, about his remarkable personality, the joy his presence communicated, and the treatments that worked wonders? After thirty years of study, Sensei was confident in his art. Just as haiku *is*, Jin Shin Jyutsu *is*. There lies in Jin Shin Jyutsu all that is Japanese. Sensei was Japanese and thus predisposed to being self-effacing and egoless. He was not offering something from himself but a gift from Japan. There was a casualness to his proposition, maybe a puckishness, too, in all events absolutely nothing condescendingly didactic. And there was no mystical fervor in Mary's consent. It was rather an expression of how open and receptive she was and how willing she was to place her trust in him. The feeling was genuine, clear, and straightforward.

Mary's "yes" to Jiro Murai was a very simple "yes." In her *Introducing Jin Shin Jyutsu IS, Book I* she would later write, "In the late 1940's, I was guided to Master Murai. At the time of our meeting I was 'searching' for that 'something' which I believe each one of us experiences at one time or another in our lifetime."

I know that kind of "yes."

More than twenty years ago, I was exploring Venice for the first time in the company of Mirella Toso, a Venetian friend of mine. In a workshop in the vicinity of San Angelo she introduced me to a bookbinder, Silvano, who was mixing glue in a pan over an old burner. I admired the marbled sheets of paper that were drying. I watched him cut and stitch paper. We were about to leave when he asked, "Would you like to make a little book with me?"

I did not immediately understand the meaning of his question, but I felt comfortable there with him, in that place and at that time. I replied, "Yes, I would. When?"

"Right now," he said.

Mirella left us. I sat down next to Silvano Gosparini and it was as if I had always known how to do what he taught me. That was the day I began learning a craft that I have continued to study ever since.

I embraced Jin Shin Jyutsu with the feeling it was a gift from life. I had my first Jin Shin Jyutsu session in the fall of 2002. I had just lost my brother. I was grieving. My brother's death had shaken us like an earthquake and plunged the family into a chaos of our own. Like the maps of Tokyo designed to help people find their way should the city be reduced to rubble, Jin Shin Jyutsu helped me find mine. Thanks to Jin Shin Jyutsu, I was able to get close to my parents who had been left stranded on an island of pain. They immediately let me sit next to them and touch them. I would place my hands on different parts of their fully dressed bodies in what soon became a ritual. Session by session, we found solace from our grief, we quieted our anger, and found a renewed sense of serenity.

I told them what Mary Burmeister said in her book *Introducing Jin Shin Jyutsu Is*: "What makes the heart beat? What makes breathing possible? What makes digestion possible? What makes a car engine start when you turn on the key? What turns the car lights on? The answer to the last two questions is simply 'the battery.' The battery is the energy source that makes everything run. And if one were to ask what is the energy source of the body, the answer would simply be: 'The battery of life'." And our hands on the "safety energy locks" function like battery cables. "Jin Shin Jyutsu is the knowing of the body's vital force of life, the source."

Mary Burmeister said, "When Master Murai put to me so simply the question, 'Would you like to study with me to take a "gift" from Japan to America?' I had no idea of the depth of its meaning at the time. So just as simply I replied, 'Yes'."

"When I attended his first lecture, I was filled with humility and awe at the 'why' I was here. My 'search' had ended and an art of living had opened for me. It was not until nearly thirty years later of continued study that the impact of the meaning in Master Murai's first greeting became a reality for me."[71]

To spread the art of Jin Shin Jyutsu throughout the world, Mary Burmeister chose instructors from many different countries. You can learn the fundamentals of Jin Shin Jyutsu in five-day classes and self-help workshops. At the end of each seminar, the instructor insists on the fact that "Jin Shin Jyutsu is" and that a person who practices it becomes the artist. The ritualized sentence is, "Be your own testimony." In effect, even if the content of the teaching does not vary, it is fascinating to hear individual instructors offer their variations on it.

In Jin Shin Jyutsu, only Jiro Murai is called Master: Murai Sensei.

Atomic Bomb
Earthquake
Pulses

Kaga now seemed a distant memory; we were very much back in Tokyo. At the supermarket, we walked past miles of shelves overflowing with soy sauce, seaweed, and rice. I stopped to watch a rice huller separate the chaff from the grain. Our basket was filling up with exquisite little tomatoes, strawberries bursting with sweetness, various kinds of sushi, and the ingredients we needed to make miso soup.

As we were leaving, Kyoko pointed out a photo booth that made pictures that showed you with a facelift. Leave it to the Japanese! The trip had to have regenerated my neurons. I had had to clear so much space in my brain for the things I was constantly discovering that the anxieties of the past had simply vanished. On our way back to the house we stopped at the post office so I could pick up some cash. Kyoko's mother had bought the land in the Ogikubo district precisely so her house would be near the post office and the train station. Neighborhoods tend to grow up around stations. Because the street had no name the post office was the landmark I used to find my way back to the house with its three tiles of Quimper faience on the facade and the numbers 3, 26, and 6 painted on them. Could this really just be coincidence? I couldn't get over it. Well before Kyoko and I met, her mother had been to France, to Quimper, which is the city in Brittany I grew up in and where my mother still lived.

Next stop, the optician's. Kyoko asked me if I still had the John Lennon glasses I had bought ten years earlier when we went strolling through the city. I always buy glasses when I travel. After that we went to a bookstore. We had ordered a magazine in which an article on Jin Shin Jyutsu was to appear and ten copies of *J'aime* (*I love*),[72] one of the children's books I wrote that had been translated into Japanese. I wanted to send a copy to all the people who had helped us. I wrote a personal note in each of the little square-shaped volumes, saying fairly much the same thing each time, thanking them with all my heart. Kyoko, who is so sweet, spent a lot of time translating and inscribing them in her beautiful calligraphy, and added a personal note of her own. The final stop was the pharmacy, to buy pain-relieving patches for my mother's arthritis. Kyoko began sending them to her regularly and a friendship grew out of it.

People on bikes sped past us. Every one looked slim and limber, and was extremely courteous, but most of the faces were hidden behind white masks that protected against the spread of infection or against pollen. (It really is time for the Japanese to discover Jin Shin Jyutsu, which views allergies as a sign of a weakened immune system.) While Kyoko was telling me that her students kept their masks on in class, which made it difficult for her to get to know them, I looked for people who weren't wearing any. I was struck by how beautiful the elderly and little children were. Ravens were cawing out their frustration at the blue fishing nets that kept garbage bags tightly sealed. In the otherwise silent megalopolis where only signs with kanji glared out from amid the jumble of electric wires, the birds made me think of Hitchcock. We stopped to admire one cherry tree after another; one more week and they would be absolutely splendid. Kyoko would later send me a few pictures with "Do you remember?" written on them. Cats were stretched out on low walls, basking in the sunlight, purring. The city was clean, absolutely clean. I finally grasped Henri Michaux's sentence, which is in every book on Japan: "The Japanese clean even the sky." I understood the uneasiness they feel when they arrive in France, an uneasiness the Japanese psychiatric world has labeled "the Paris syndrome." I also realized that kneeling down to roll up your futon, storing it in the closet, sweeping the tatami with a rice-straw broom with a handle much shorter than those on our brooms and that forces you to bend over, and making sure the table and cushions are perfectly centered... all these little movements that are performed mindfully constitute daily gymnastic exercises that are excellent for muscles and joints. In 1585, Luis Frois wrote, "At home, a gentleman would consider it shameful to sweep out his bedroom. Japanese lords do it willingly and are happy to."[73]

東京
Tokyo

It was Sunday. We were on the bus to Nagatacho, the city district with government offices, to meet up with Kyoko's friend Kazumi for a demonstration against the repeal of article 9. Prime Minister Shinzo Abe was so concerned with China's enormous power and North Korea's unpredictability that he wanted to restore Japan's military sovereignty.

The vote on Article 9 of the Japanese Constitution was a major moment in the history of modern Japan. The law was passed on November 3, 1946, during US occupation, and went into effect on May 3, 1947.

It decrees that Japan will never go to war.

Tokyo has been leveled twice: following an earthquake in 1923 and from American bombing raids in 1945.

At a time when there were no hospitals left standing and no medications, Jiro Murai had nonetheless been able to bring relief, comfort, and encouragement to the ailing simply by placing his hands on their bodies or holding their fingers. The months of immense suffering had provided him with countless opportunities to experiment with his treatments.

As we frequently see in Japanese films, the Japanese are reluctant to touch each other when they express their feelings, yet they have no qualms about getting a massage. *Teate* (to touch) means to treat.

手当
Care

In 1923 the city had been the capital of the Empire for slightly more than fifty years and had a population of two million. (Paris had three million, New York, five, London seven.) There were still many wooden buildings dating back to the time the city was named Edo, and which a Lumière brothers' camera operator filmed in 1898. They stood in stark contrast to the Western style headquarters of fast-growing corporations. Bridges were built with steel or Renaissance style stone, like the Nihonbashi Bridge near the fish market. A new train station had opened in 1914. Samurai, who no longer carried swords, moved about on orange-colored electric tramways.

September 1. It was 11:58 am when the first tremor hit. It was followed by a second one, and then a third that wreaked havoc throughout the city. A raging typhoon spread fire everywhere, setting kimonos aflame. Panic-stricken crowds of people tried to flee, but there was no access to any of the waterways. Stunned Tokyoites witnessed the total destruction of their city's historical center. Of the Ginza district there remained nothing but rubble. The train station collapsed, bridges went up in flames. The toll was tremendous: a hundred and five thousand victims in the space of three days and two nights. The Great Kanto Earthquake would leave people profoundly traumatized. During that September of 1923, a million and a half homeless people roamed Ueno Park in search of their loved ones. The then French ambassador, Paul Claudel, was struck by how calm and orderly people were. "Not a single person complained," he wrote. "You weren't supposed to bother your neighbors. Everyone was supposed to remain calm."[74] There was a shortage of everything. Tokyo had been reduced to a gigantic shantytown. "Even though our houses have been burned to the ground, we are still Tokyoites," the Japanese asserted and started re-building immediately.[75] Walking through Ueno Park, I saw homeless people sitting cross-legged on pieces of cardboard, as if meditating, their shoes neatly set out next to them.

By 1930, just seven years after the earthquake, a new Tokyo had arisen, and Japan was on its way to becoming the world's third greatest power. Paul Claudel remained highly impressed with the resilience of the Japanese.

Tokyo was the target of American bombing raids from February to June 1945. On the night of March 9, the city was subjected to a deluge of high explosive, incendiary bombs that killed nearly one hundred thousand people. Kenneth Werrell called it "one of the deadliest airstrikes of all time."[76] During the summer of 1945, night after night, cities went up in smoke. Sixty-eight Japanese cities were targeted, two, Hiroshima and Nagasaki, with atom bombs. Kyoto was spared because it is a cultural heritage site, but more than forty percent of every major Japanese city was destroyed, and for Tokyo the figure was sixty. The loss of human life was devastating, the material damage catastrophic, the psychological consequences… incalculable. The Tokyo trial, the Asian equivalent of the Nuremberg trial, ran from 1946 to 1948, after which Japan committed to pacifism.

In Alain Resnais and Marguerite Duras' *Hiroshima mon amour* (*Hiroshima, My Love*), a Japanese man asks a French woman,

"What did Hiroshima mean to you?" She replies, "It meant the end of the war. Astonishment that they had dared. Astonishment that they had succeeded. And for us, the beginning of a fear we had never known."

The Children of Nagasaki

In 1983, Keisuke Kinoshita made the first film about the atomic bombing of Nagasaki. He based it on the life of Takashi Nagai. The film opens with archival footage of Pope John-Paul II addressing a Christian congregation during his visit to Urakami Cathedral in 1981: "War is man's doing, war destroys human lives, war means death… Hiroshima and Nagasaki are proof of our misfortune… forever, their names must be honored … To remember the past is to engage in the future."

The film underscores our obligation to pass things on to future generations.

A new kind of bomb had been dropped on the city. "The city instantly became a sea of fire. It might have been an atom bomb."

These are the words of Dr. Nagai, a survivor now living in a doomsday landscape. He has invited to his home students who have just returned from the front lines. He shows them the report he has just written on the atom bomb.

"It was said that after a nuclear attack neither animal nor vegetal life would exist for another seventy-five years, but just three weeks later I spotted an ant colony very close to the epicenter. A month later, there were earthworms, and rats running wild everywhere."

"What you're saying is reassuring," a student says.

"Just as I feared," Nagai retorts. "There is a problem in feeling reassured. It is as if a nuclear bomb were not that serious. Within a thousand-yard radius from the epicenter death was instantaneous; within five hundred yards, bellies burst open and guts spilled out; at seven hundred yards, heads with their eyes popped out were ripped off bodies. Our neighborhood shelter was six hundred yards from the center. With the exception of one child at the back, everyone was killed. My mother-in-law lost eleven relatives: two of her daughters, her brother-in-law, his wife, and their children."

Like Jiro Murai, Takashi Nagai was born into a family of physicians and samurai. His father, Noboro Nagai, practiced Ranpo (Western) medicine, his grandfather, Fumitika Nagai, Kampo (traditional) medicine. In April 1928, Nagai enrolled at the medical school of Nagasaki University. In the midst of his studies, he embarked on a spiritual journey that led him from Shintoism to Atheism and then to Catholicism. In January 1933 he did his military service in Manchuria where he was in charge of sanitary services. The acts of violence and brutality the Japanese perpetrated on the Chinese civilian population left him terribly shaken. He turned to the Bible and read Blaise Pascal's Pensées, "There is enough light for those who wish to see and enough darkness for those who are of a contrary disposition."[77]

Up until his death on May 1, 1951, Dr. Nagai never stopped writing, nor did his son, who became a journalist, stop writing about him.[78]

In 1946 Jiro Murai met his American disciple, Mary Iino Burmeister, a year after Japan surrendered.

For thirty-three years, Murai Sensei had been carrying out research with the aim of giving Jin Shin Jyutsu back to the world. For thirty-three years, in a country ravaged by war and chaos, he had worked relentlessly to retrieve from ancestral memory the forgotten art of harmonizing energy.

Where had he lived during those thirty-three years? With whom? What did he live on?

In Haruki Kato's book, I learned that Murai had been banished by his parents. The idea of banishment was commonplace in Japanese culture. It meant cut off from "family" and thus deprived of financial support. To further his knowledge of the circulation of fluids, Murai frequented a slaughterhouse where, for five yen, he could buy ox heads immediately after the animals were killed. He also befriended crematorium employees who let him secretly study corpses just before they were cremated. At the time, only the outcast *burakumin* were allowed to touch the dead. Did he carry out dissections, which only certified physicians were allowed to do? Was he turned in to the authorities? Was he caught red-handed? Arrested? Tried? Haruki Kato said that Jiro Murai did many things that went well beyond what ordinary people could ever imagine or fathom. He was a free spirit and fearless. Nothing could keep him from pursuing his quest.

Denied an allowance, penniless, he went and knocked on his niece's door. When did that happen? Before 1923? His niece was studying to be a doctor. She gave up her studies to help him in his research and remained with him until his death. Her name was Toku, which means "virtue." It would be so nice to know more about her. At that time, it took a remarkable woman to pursue medical studies, which was true not just in Japan but everywhere else in the world as well. She had to have come from a very progressive family of renowned physicians.

In 1960, Jiro Murai died of kidney cancer. It might have resulted from the many dietary restrictions to which he subjected his body as part of his research. By listening to his own pulses he had predicted his death two years prior to the event. Sadaki Kato was convinced that the cause of death was unrelated to the ailment that had made doctors declare him terminally ill in 1912. In Yojiro Takita's *Departures* (2008), we learn about funeral rites in Japan through the main character, a cellist who has found employment in a funeral home. Following a family meal, everyone kneels on a tatami to witness the cleansing of the departed. The cleansing is carried out with meticulous care, every movement gentle and measured so as to help family and friends deal with the final separation. It is a rite of purification, not unlike the baths given newborns, but intended here to prepare the deceased for their journey into the afterlife. There is no unseemly display of flesh. The naked body is concealed beneath an artfully arranged kimono. Before the body is placed in the coffin, the undertaker makes a suggestion. "You might want to run a cloth over his face to say goodbye." Then, just before closing the coffin he adds, "Please join hands to help make his departure a peaceful one."

Jin Shin Jyutsu recognizes 72 pulses.

During my third session with Sadaki Kato he listened to my pulses as he had done previously, then chose to work on the 10 flow and the kidney flow. We had begun to know each other well. He informed me of what he had sensed. A practitioner listens to the pulses on each wrist twice, to get the superficial pulse and the deep one. When the body is in balance, the right and left pulses are in harmony. If there is imbalance, one of the two or both will be rapid, uneven, heavy, chaotic, feeble, or silent, indicating disharmony. The superficial pulse corresponds to descending energy (the energy we receive from the sky) and the deep pulse to ascending energy (the energy we receive from the Earth). The right wrist speaks of the present, the left of the past, of our genetic heritage. A practitioner places the fingers of his left hand on the patient's right wrist and vice versa. Under the left index, he listens to the large intestine, the lungs, and the second depth; under the right index, to the small intestine, the heart, and the fifth depth; under the left middle finger, to the stomach, the spleen, and the first depth; under the right middle finger, to the gall bladder, the liver, and the third depth; under the left ring finger, to the diaphragm, the umbilicus, and the sixth depth; and under the right ring finger, to the bladder, the kidney, and the fourth depth.

Rakugo Theater
Ginkgo Nuts
Laughter

There always comes a time when Kyoko and I have to part ways.

At train stations, my rail pass gets me in through a special entrance. I show the pass, I bow, I am invited to proceed, they bow back. I am a foreigner, a *gaijin*, a "person from elsewhere." The *gaijin* that I am is highly impressed by how fluid and civil life is. People line up for the subway or the train, without pushing or shoving. Instead of the ambient fear cities tend to generate, there is a sense of being "embraced," as François Laplantine put it in *Le Japon ou le sens des extrêmes* (*Japan or the Land of Extremes*). He added, "It is difficult to imagine a society in which you feel as appreciated and pampered as you do here. In France, people often feel they are on their own."[79] Here, there is a groove cut into the ticket counter to keep your umbrella from falling. When I walk into a department store, a young woman hands me a plastic sleeve for my wet umbrella. When I sit down at a counter to order a cup of coffee, the waiter rolls over a little basket for my purse. In Japan, God is in the details. In France, the details are the devil's playground! In response to my quip, Kyoko cast an impish smile at me. But later, in Shibuya, she pointed out a small sign at the foot of an escalator. It said that it was illegal to take pictures up a woman's skirt or to grope a woman's behind. "They have to have everything spelled out for them," she said, with a hint of exasperation more typical of the French, "even to loosen their tie when it's hot."

I could no longer ride the subway without imagining an earthquake. The train we were on was speeding underground towards Asakusa. Sadaki Kato, whom we had gone to see for a third session upon our return from Kaga, said that Asakusa is where Jiro Murai probably spent his youth, carousing and ruining his health. As described in Yasunari Kawabata's novel *The Scarlet Gang of Asakusa* (1930),[80] it is a district that still has remnants of the capital dating to the Edo period when there were booths of all sorts, performers, dancers, geishas, tightrope walkers, and so on. Watch out for the bike-taxi! I was taking a picture of a young woman standing in a doorway with an owl perched on the sleeve of her yellow oilskin. A short distance from Ueno Park, on the banks of the Sumida River, at the end of Kappabashi Street, stand Senso-ji and, next to it, a five-story pagoda. Senso-ji is dedicated to the goddess Bodhisattva Kannon. It is Tokyo's oldest Buddhist temple, first built in 645 and then rebuilt in 1958. Its portal is known as Kaminari-mon, "Thunder Gate," and there is a massive red paper lantern, the largest in Japan, hanging down from it. Visitors gorge themselves on rice balls stuffed with red bean paste. Was Jiro Murai addicted to these little delicacies? We visited the temple, bowing respectfully, and left offerings. It was not far from there to the Shinto temple, so we headed over and went through the same routine: visiting, bowing, making an offering. Then we took a short walk around the grounds, a little gem of an oasis in the midst of skyscrapers with the Sky Tree Tower grandest of all. We came out onto a street lined with shops that made you want to go in and buy everything. We stopped at a kimono shop, and a ceramic shop, and a kitchenware shop, and a broom shop. This last one was a delightful place with a thousand and one brooms and brushes of all kinds. We lingered there for quite a while. "Placing a broom upside down near the door means you're anxious to see your guests leave," Kyoko told me. We left with a mushroom brush, a toothbrush, a hairbrush, a body brush, and a bamboo brush for frying pans… as well as the address of a good restaurant with the best buckwheat noodles in town. They served us buckwheat tofu, fava beans, ginkgo nuts, every dish a savory delight. What a treat!

There were pictures on the wall of their regulars, all of them actors from a *Rakugo* theater.

"Want to go?"

We got to the theater at 2:30. The show runs all day long. The theater was packed and smelled of street food. Everyone was laughing. People were coming and going. We made our way along a wall and found seats. *Rakugo* is a form of comedy that dates back to the Edo period. The profession is hereditary and performers take on the name of their mentors. There are no sets and no music. The performer is dressed in a kimono and sits seiza-style on a cushion. His only prop is a fan. The story he tells can be long and complicated, or short and simple; or it can be satirical or political. Whatever it is, it has to have a funny punch line. Everybody was howling; Kyoko, too. The performer, whose name was written on an easel in kanji, was telling the story of a man who practices acupuncture on his asthmatic cat. It was as if it was intended for me. Since I could not partake of the gaiety, I tried to take a picture. When I raised my iPhone, the woman next to me tapped me on the hand. I quickly put the phone away. So, no pictures allowed, apparently. Laughter is good for your health. All of the old-timers there knew that. They had come to have a good laugh the way other people go for a massage.

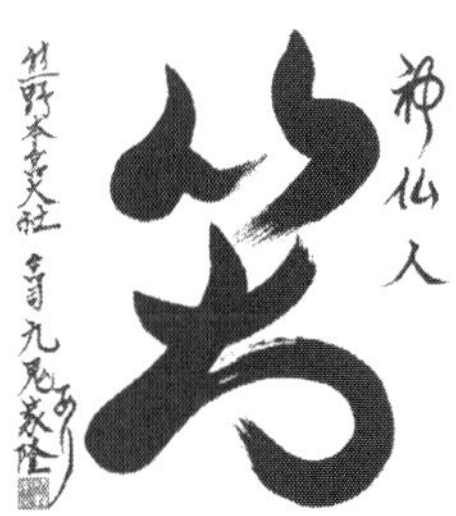

The kanji for laughter; calligraphy done by a priest at the Kumamo Hongu Taisha Temple

Did the inspiration for the 15 flow come to Jiro Murai in one of these *Rakugo* theaters? Safety energy locks 15 are located on either side of the groin. Holding them helps you relax. It is the comedian's flow, renewed intelligence, and the laughter that cleanses the subconscious. It helps alleviate issues with the heart and the brain. As they say, laughter is the best medicine. You should always have in mind something to laugh about.

Tsujido
Mountain and Sea
Testament

I looked for Jiro Murai in Kaga; he was in Tokyo. I looked for him in Tokyo; he was in Tsujido.

It was a beautiful spring morning and there we were, at Shinjuku Station, boarding the train for Tsujido. I had tried to find out what Tokyo neighborhood Murai Sensei lived in when Haruki Kato was his student and, true to form, learned that he had lived in Tsujido, and in a beautiful house with his niece, Toku.

"Papa Kato," as Kyoko called Haruki, might have occasionally visited him there between 1953 and 1960.

Jiro Murai ended his life very much as he had started it, between the mountains and the sea: in Kaga, between the Sea of Japan and Mount Haku; in Tsujido, between the Pacific and Mount Fuji. Tsujido is about an hour from the heart of Tokyo. Its train station was destroyed twice, during the 1923 earthquake and then by bombing raids in 1945. After Tsujido, the train continues on to the small seaside resort of Kamakura, the de facto capital of Japan between 1185 and 1333 that is famous for a monumental statue of the Buddha that has embodied Zen Buddhism for more than eight centuries. Filmmaker Yasujiro Ozu had a predilection for the region, just as he loved to include trains and train stations in his films. Once a month, Jiro Murai took that train to Tokyo, to teach and give treatments.

Did his niece, Toku, bear any resemblance to Yasujiro Ozu's muse, the actress Setsuko Hara?

Was their everyday life similar to that of the father and daughter in *Late Spring*? The Japanese phrase "*ishin-denshin*" expresses the ideal relationship between people who are so close that neither words nor gestures are necessary.

Every significant Japanese author of the 20th century spent time in the Kamakura region. Did Jiro Murai meet Natsume Soseki, Osamu Dazai, Ryunosuke Akutagawa, Yukio Mishima, Sanjugo Naoki, Masaoka Shiki, Akiko Yosano, or Yasunari Kawabata?

Wealthy Tokyoites used to come to Tsujido and the surrounding area for their health and the sanatoriums here. Even the Prime Minister has a villa here. Jiro Murai might well have had an affluent clientele and built a network of relations, and through them gained an introduction to the Imperial family, whom we know he treated.

It was also in Tsujido that destitute families were lodged in subsidized housing after the war.

We took a bus to the beach.

At the top of a building, among many signs in kanji, I saw "Salon de Mine." Kyoko and I were delighted. Kyoko calls me Mine. Daniel started calling me Mine when we first met and I have used it to sign my children's books, some of which have been translated into Japanese. To add a touch of nobility to the monosyllabic name – spelled by some with an Asian twist, Minh – I added an *n*, like the French writer Colette's Minne. For Kyoko, "Salon de Mine" was a sign. Throughout our journey, the feeling that we were accompanied and guided never left us.

A long white sandy beach awaited, a surfer's paradise.

I spent much of my childhood building sandcastles on a beach just like this one and much of my adolescence watching sunsets and dreaming about love, and my youth, reading the complete works of my literary mentor, Georges Perros.

Jiro Murai lived in this landscape that I know so well. He is bound to have taken long walks on the beach and to have gazed at the moon. (Today, October 3rd, the moon is supposed to be at its most beautiful. Kyoko would send me pictures).

It was on that beach that Jiro Murai shared thoughts with Mary Burmeister that she would later pass on to her students:

> No bird who flies on his own wings flies too high.
> You are a star, I am a star, we are the stars.
> We are the creation. A replica of the cosmos.
> Life is comical and simple.
> The body mirrors our thoughts. What's wrong is in us, and only in us.
> All misfortune is the product of ignorance.
> Drop the shoulders and breathe!
> Look until you can hear. Listen until you can see.
> Where you are is your home.
> You are your best friend.
> You were born perfect. You are perfection. Be perfect everyday.
> Don't analyze, harmonize. Be the testimony, not the critic.
> You are your own teacher.
> Without imagination one gets nowhere.
> Never forget to laugh![81]

On that beach, he would have prepared the lectures that inspired the talks Mary would give:

"Introducing Jin Shin Jyutsu 'is,' is only to awaken our awareness as to what 'being' is. It is simply the getting to know (help) myself."

"Through Jin Shin Jyutsu our awareness is awakened to the simple fact that all that is needed for harmony and balance (rhythm with the universe) physically, mentally, emotionally, digestively and spiritually is within myself. Through this awareness the feeling of complete peace, serenity, security, the oneness within is evident. No person, situation or thing can take these away from myself. All fears (the basis of all disharmony) begin to dissipate one by one and all unnecessary burdens are unloaded from our shoulders to make way for the complete within and without. There is no room for feelings of competition and comparison in our everyday living. There is only the present state of be-ing, which already is our 'past' and the foundation of our 'future'."

We stopped at the surfers' kiosk on Surfers Street. In Jiro Murai's lifetime it was called Showa Street, after the Emperor who reigned from 1926 to 1989. Before the tsunami, there were twenty-five surfers' shops; only two are left. Since 2011, the price of buildable coastal land has dropped thirty percent. While Kyoko was chatting away, the image of *The Wave* came back to me. We had seen Hokusai's (1760-1849) woodblock print the day before, in the Ota Memorial Museum of Art. There are two small boats in the trough of a gigantic circular wave, and two men, smaller still, trying to steer their way through the raging sea. Far in the distance, a small triangle appears against a leaden sky: Mount Fuji. The print is one of a series of thirty-six views of Mount Fuji done by Hokusai between 1831 and 1834.

The thirty-six views of Mount Fuji!

The Thirty-Six Immortals of Poetry! They were a group of remarkable poets that included three women, one of them famous for her beauty, who were active during the Heian period. (The women used their father's or husband's name, or a pseudonym.) The group created "the laws of thirty-six." Basho said, "The great poet takes thirty-six steps. Poetry is composed of thirty-six poems. The poet should never look back. When you move forward, your heart is regenerated and eventually moving forward is all you think of."[82]

Haiku master Basho came here and celebrated Mount Fuji.

Coming into view
Especially at this hour
Mount Fuji in May

– Basho

For Hokusai, as for Basho, nature is not just the world outside. It encompasses all cosmic creation through which life flows and transmigrates. In Japan, naturally, 36 is an auspicious number.

In Jin Shin Jyutsu we speak of thirty-six breaths. It is an exercise that regulates and deepens the breath. The thirty-six-breath practice is quite simple: all you need to do is fold your arms across your chest and place your hands under your armpits, where safety energy locks 26 are located. Then you start breathing, counting each breath: 1, I breathe out, I breathe in; 2, I breathe out, I breathe in… thirty-six times or in groups of nine. This will restore balance in all the inner functions of the body.

"Exhale – Unload all dirt, dust, and greasy grime.
(FEAR – False Evidence Appearing Real.)
Inhale – Receive the purified Cosmic Energy.
(FUN – Fulfillment, Understanding, No-thing.)"

The French instructor Nathalie Max said that the first time she performed this exercise she immediately experienced a sensation that changed her life.

I like to do it with children whenever I visit classrooms to show them my books. Together, with our arms crossed and our hands under our armpits, we take nine breaths, which is just long enough for them to let go of one activity and be ready to engage in another.

津波
Tsunami

There will very likely be another earthquake in Tokyo some time in the next thirty years, Kyoko said. She added, "Or so they've been saying for the last thirty years!" In Japan, nature can be extremely violent. The 2011 earthquake was deadly and devastating. It happened on March 11. Kyoko was in Tokyo; I was in Paris. The news channels flooded the airwaves with apocalyptic images. We were worried about our Japanese friends.

In the French translation of Yoko Tawada's *After Fukushima. Reflections on a Culture in Turmoil* (*Journal des jours tremblants après Fukushima*), I underlined the following entry: "March 13, 2011. As children we were taught to remain calm in the event of natural catastrophe. Now, whenever I hear the words 'natural catastrophe', I feel very calm … My heartbeat slows as if I had taken a tranquilizer."[83]

The ocean air had made us hungry. There were two bars; we chose the one that was empty but welcoming in appearance. They had little curried fish sandwiches and coffee. Our host told us he had seen Mount Fuji when he woke up that morning. Here, Mount Fuji is the main topic of conversation and the subject of countless pictures on Facebook. The sacred mountain speaks and gives the weather forecast for the day. I was drawn to the counter, the way Geppetto was drawn to the piece of wood that became Pinocchio. Our host was happy to tell us that it was cypress wood and came from a bar that was being razed. Before that, it had been a pillar in a historical house. Was there a historical house nearby that was open to the public? Our host quickly called a friend to come and show us around in his pedicab. In his charming Osaka accent, the driver described the writer Toson Shimazaki's house (1872-1943) in Oiso. Shimazaki was a poet, essayist, and novelist and is considered one of the founders of Japanese naturalism. His fourth novel, *Shinsei* (*New Life*) is an autobiographical account of his scandal-provoking liaison with his niece Komako. The writer fled to France when she became pregnant and remained there until 1914.[84]

"Did Jiro Murai love Toku in the same way?" Kyoko mused. We were too late for the last visit, but on a panel at the entrance we learned that the writer had died at seventy-one, while his wife was reading one of his manuscripts to him. In one breath he said, "The wind is chilly" and then he was gone.

Cyclecabin, the pedi-cab operator, was pedaling his way between cars. We were on our way to Enoshima. He, too, had been to France, to Paris, and especially knew the Cour Carrée in the Louvre because he generally went there for Fashion Week. Before starting his small pedi-cab business he had worked in the ready-to-wear industry. We chatted about fashion. My relationship with Japan started when I was a journalist for *Marie-Claire* and helped start *Marie-Claire Japan*.

I mentioned my favorite fashion designer, Yohji Yamamoto. Cyclecabin and I are now Facebook friends.

He dropped us off on Enoshima Island, the equivalent of France's Mont Saint-Michel. The temple was dedicated to Benzaiten, one of the Seven Gods of Fortune. The goddess, also known as Benten, is at the heart of the legend of the island.

Benten and the Enoshima Dragon

Once upon a time, long, long ago, there was a dragon, the most terrible of dragons, who used to devour children. A dragon this cruel, Benton thought, must he unhappy. The goddess went to the monster's lair, lifted it up above the sea, and turned it into Enoshima Island. She then came down from the heavens and approached the dragon with a beguiling smile. "No one can live without affection. Let's get married! Let's have children! You will love them, I know it! The dragon agreed and ever since that day calm has prevailed on the coast of Enoshima.

In her introductory work on Jin Shin Jyutsu, Mary Burmeister said, "Jin Shin Jyutsu is a 'built-in' simple art of living. Getting to know (help) myself. It is an art and not a technique. An art requires much understanding and is creative, which is simple. A technique requires much effort in memorizing and is imitative, has limitations and is competitive, therefore, complex."[85]

Ise Jingu
A Humble Dwelling
The Bonze

I began writing as soon as I got back to France. Japan, Jin Shin Jyutsu, and Jiro Murai were with me everyday. As always, Kyoko arrived at the end of August, her suitcase filled with gifts she would take out, one by one, at various points during her stay. The last one she gave us, the evening before she left, was an etching on a red background with a well-known sentence by Natsume Soseki, in English: *I am a cat, I have yet no name.*[86] I hung it on the red wall in our living room and read it everyday. I want to learn to say it in Japanese: *Wagahai wa neki derau. Namae ha mada na.*

Jiro Murai is a cat. Every time I got hold of him, he slipped away. Whenever I do the main central exercise, my cat Perlette jumps on me, lies down, and stretches. When I type, she snuggles against my shoulder and hops onto the keyboard. Jiro Murai has made a place for himself inside me. He has changed the ozone in my home. He is a healer-cat.

Kyoko gave me a volume of Basho's haiku in Japanese. The poet-traveler had been our guide, illuminating our path like a beacon.

Basho said, "Haiku IS."

Jiro Murai said, "Jin Shin Jyutsu IS."

A haiku is a game with numbers.

So is Jin Shin Jyutsu.

Jiro Murai is a poet and, like all poets, he is attuned to the stars.

Kyoko had brought rice flour with her and used some to make us zucchini, eggplant, carrot and onion tempura. This was on a wonderful summer day in the mountains, after we had come back from a long hike. While she cooked, I read aloud *The Pillow Book* by the 10th century poetess Sei-Shonagon: "In the spring, at dawn, I love to watch the hazy sky gradually brighten, while wisps of purple clouds trail over the mountaintops."[87]

We were planning our next trip, for 2018. We would go in the spring when the cherry trees were in bloom. I wanted to dream in a haze of cherry blossoms, *hanagasumi*. And I was determined to convince Kyoko to go on the Shinto pilgrimage at Ise Jingu.

On an afternoon in March 2018, one year from the start of our first trip, we left Tokyo for Ise. By bullet train the trip takes three hours. It took us four. My rail pass was not valid for all trains; I could not travel on the Kin Tetsu line. Booking our tickets online turned out to be impossible. We had to buy tickets for Nagoya at the station in Tokyo, then tickets for Ise in Nagoya. When a train reaches the end of the line, all the seats are turned around to face in the direction it will be heading next.

At that time of year, there are no hotel vacancies. We had made a reservation in an inn that offered yoga and meditation and did not ask for a deposit. I could tell that Kyoko was worried. The name of the guesthouse was Gukyo An. Kyoko finally revealed that *gu* means "idiot," *kyo* means "crazy," and *an* means "humble lodging." She had called the inn twice: once from Nagoya and then again from the station in Ise to get directions for the taxi driver. It was 8:00 pm and pitch black when we pulled open the door to Gukyo An. It was beyond humble, it was downright primitive, and was run by two men. The one who greeted us looked us over in amusement. All the rooms were booked, there, too. Without knowing it, we had reserved a tent!

A tent by the side of a mountain stream! Kyoko and I avoided looking at each other. I was the one who had made the reservation. The French love to camp out, our host declared as he zipped open the ridge tent with one hand while holding a flashlight in the other. This was going to be a long night! What's more, there were no restaurants in the area where we could spend a quiet evening, just a convenience store. We sat at the kitchen table in the inn and ate our ketchup omelet in its plastic container. Never had I eaten so poorly in the Land of the Rising Sun. A young woman and two children had just arrived in a taxi. They were going to sleep in a van next to our tent. Well, if monkeys attack, they'll be there to defend us! Her children were having a grand time. They all went out as soon as the kids got out of the bath. The bathroom was right next to the kitchen; it smelled of grease… and the kitchen smelled of soap. As we ate our pitiful dinner, other lodgers kept passing by. However seedy the place was, it at least had a bath. For the first time I found Kyoko a little squeamish. No, she said, we would not be taking a bath that evening. We would just brush our teeth. Outside, the air was cold and damp. We decided to hang out on the tatami in the main room as long as possible. I knelt; Kyoko knelt. Steam was rising from a teapot on the brazier. A few guests came in and went up to their rooms. Lucky devils! The innkeeper was sitting cross-legged focused on his computer. His associate kept bringing him large glasses of warm saké. The decoration was strange: a stuffed owl perched on a console table, a shrine framing the portrait of an old bearded master, a skeleton in a corner, and right next to me a black and gold lacquered mask.

"That is Ko-Shinto! He who opens the way," our host explained, "a god more ancient than Amaterasu, the god I am descended from."

The conversation took off from there and never waned. It was as if our host had been waiting for us to come.

He introduced himself. We were in the home of a bonze, Genryu, the first dragon!

I took out my notepad and started to interview him.

He had a sense of humor. He was friendly, lighthearted, and talkative. "Even compared to other bad bonzes," he admitted, "I am one of the worst."

Genryu was born in 1974. He came from a poor family, dirt poor. His life's ambition was to make a lot of money, by any means necessary. He joined the *yakuzas*, the Japanese mafia, and soon rose through the ranks. A life in the underworld and a life of luxury. It was easy to imagine him in a white suit and pointed shoes, drinking champagne in a limousine with tinted windows, sitting alongside Ginza's most gorgeous prostitutes. He was not even thirty when he was arrested and tried for murder. It was a crime, he said, he had not committed intentionally. He was convicted and spent two years in solitary confinement, in a cell the size of three and half tatamis. He never saw the light of day and had no one to talk to. On Friday, they served curry. That was the only thing that prevented him from completely losing the sense of time. He wanted to die and he didn't want to die. He was afraid he was going crazy. He started meditating, doing *zazen*, and reading the Bible and other sacred texts, and one day he became enlightened. He immediately wrote to more than a dozen religious leaders. Not one of them responded. He was thoroughly discouraged and decided that much of religion was a lie. On his release from prison, he cut ties with the *yakuzas*, putting his life in danger. Having gone through that, nothing would ever scare him again. He took off his shirt to show us his tattoos. (I learned that day that people with tattoos are not allowed in public baths). Genryu then went to Myanmar to study the Buddha's teachings. Buddha, he was pleased to remind us, was not a Buddhist. He also practiced waterfall meditation for an hour at a time back then, and developed an interest in Origuchi

Nobuo's school of Shintoism. Then he happened upon a picture in the press of Sharbat Gula, the Afghan Girl with green eyes. He was overcome with emotion. Whatever it was in his heart that had been holding him back burst open.

"How many years of study do you need to become a bonze?"

"Five hundred! At least!"

We laughed.

Did he have memories of his previous reincarnations?

He remembered quite clearly having been Indian. Now his vocation was to encourage people who had once been hoodlums to meditate.

How much did he meditate per day?

Ah, that was indeed the question! Meditation permeates every moment of the day. And be careful of meditation that is overly spiritual. He pointed to a round figurine, a Daruma doll that is considered a talisman of good luck in Japan. Daruma is modeled after Bodhidharma, the founder, legend has it, of Zen Buddhism. He has neither arms nor legs, having lost them when his blood ceased circulating after nine years of constant meditation.

I noticed a tear-off calendar on a shelf. It was open to the 8th of the month. His disciple laughed and tore off the page. The days had gone by unnoticed. It was the Chinese calendar. With the number 8 came another connection between us. Genryu pointed out that when 3 integrated its shadow it became 8. And 3 is an important number, because it helps create relationships.

I shifted my focus to his companion. After studying law, he had traveled all over the world, had worked in a casino in Macao, and walked the pilgrimage trail to Santiago de Compostela. But now that he was with Genryu, he had no desire to go elsewhere.

"In Ise," he said, "the journey comes to us."

I had another burning question.

"Why the skeleton?"

I was so pleased to learn that Genryu was a healer. He had studied chiropractic and also did massages. I spoke to him about Jin Shin Jyutsu and told him that I had come to retrace Jiro Murai's steps and eventually write about it.

"My turn to ask questions," he said suddenly. I closed my notepad and looked straight at him. He asked, "Where is God?"

He did not ask who is God.

"Where is God?"

I placed my hand on my heart. "God is within me."

Genryu bowed, as if having received my response as a gift.

As we were getting up to say goodnight and go out to the tent, Genryu startled us by taking us in his arms and hugging us. His hands rested a while on my safety energy locks 2, which are located in the lower back, on either side of the pelvis. Safety energy lock 2 is the body's chiropractor; it works to keep our skeleton in alignment. It helps with balance and allows us to adapt to any situation. It deals with breathing in. It is the wisdom that believes in mankind. Safety energy lock 2 teaches us to receive and to let go of our fears.

The night would be eventful and feel both short and long. It was filled with uncontrollable laughter. We laughed at finding ourselves with such primitive accommodations when we had been dreaming of a luxury hotel with an onsen, like the one we had the previous year in Kaga. We laughed at having repentant hoodlums for innkeepers. We laughed imagining the look on Daniel's face when he got the picture of Genryu's tattoos with the caption, "Don't worry, sweetheart, the innkeeper only used to be a *yakuza*; now he is a bonze." We laughed imagining everything our friends would read into the way the bonze hugged us. We laughed imagining a monkey running off with Kyoko's shoes that she had left outside the tent. We laughed because there was laughter coming out of one of the inn windows, from four young women who had come to Ise to celebrate their graduation. We laughed trying to conceive of this adventure happening in France. Wouldn't we have been terrified at the thought of spending a night in the middle of a forest near a shack with two ex-cons? But here, we both agreed, there was nothing to fear. We slept fully dressed, with just a survival blanket separating us from the ground. What happened to the futon? It had been hot when we left Tokyo; we came that close to leaving without coats. To keep warm, we kept moving closer to each other, and at one point the center pole almost collapsed. I was so grateful for Kyoko's foresightedness. She pulled heating pads out of her bag and I slipped some between my two pairs of socks to keep my feet warm. They were little pockets filled with coal, and I had no idea how they worked. The Japanese put heating pads on the sensitive areas of their bodies for all sorts of reasons: bellyaches, backaches, tendinitis…

The next morning, with our hearts cleansed by laughter, our minds emptied of all points of reference, and our bodies freed of our habitual need for comfort, we set out on the pilgrimage.

"We have somewhat met Jiro," Kyoko said. "Don't you think?"

Jiro Murai bequeathed his work on Jin Shin Jyutsu to Ise Jingu, also known as the Ise Grand Shrine, in the city of Ise, in Mie Prefecture. It is the largest Shinto shrine in Japan. That day, we had a 4 o'clock appointment at the temple library, which houses in perpetuity all books on Shintoism. The librarian came to greet us in a wheelchair. We took off our shoes and followed him into an empty study room. Kyoko explained what I was looking for. He went back out immediately. I assumed that the collection would be computerized and categorized by author and subject. There were age-old volumes hand-stitched in the Japanese style in display cases. Was that what the notebooks Jiro Murai entrusted to the library looked like? The librarian came back.

There was nothing on Jiro Murai.

And nothing on Jin Shin Jyutsu, either.

I felt like laughing. Kyoko did too. I absolutely did not want to leave the place. I sat down at a table and took out my notepad. We learned that the library had initially been located down by the river, under the bridge that leads to the pilgrimage site. In 1923, it was heavily damaged by a flood that destroyed many of its holdings. Could Jiro Murai's notebooks have been carried off by the current? Later, on my return from Japan, Inger Van Dobben would give me a book barely sixty pages long, small enough to put in your pocket but which contains all of Jin Shin Jyutsu, with columns of numbers from 1 to 26 and next to them just a few words: "left, right, left flow, right flow." I now wonder if Jiro Murai did not entrust the library with similar-sized documents, so unassuming they might have been overlooked. I handed my card to the librarian and Kyoko wrote her email address on it. Was there any chance he could keep on searching? Or could he let us know us if someone else came along asking for the same materials?

Before leaving I made one more request.

Would it be possible to have a look at the *Kojiki*?

The librarian handed us a copy of an edition from 1426.

What about the scrolls from 712? Were they kept here?

There are no scrolls from 712. The first edition of the first book dates from 1374.

Ah, Japan!

Pilgrimage
The House of Amaterasu
Secret no Secret

Throngs of pilgrims have been coming to Ise for more than two thousand years. In days gone by, a person who could not go there himself would send his dog. I have no doubt that Jiro Murai crossed over the Ujibashi bridge, bowed in front of the first torii and then the second and, just as we did, followed a stream of pilgrims down the rocky trails that lead to the heart of the sacred forest, all the way to the shrine dedicated to the goddess Amaterasu. In the history of Japan, Amaterasu Omikami is none other than the Sun goddess from whom the Imperial family is descended. The *Kojiki* tells us that the gods are much like us; they are not superior to us, and we are both of the same essence. Amaterasu is accompanied by hundreds of other deities. She is worshipped through rituals that center on the activities of daily life and vary with the seasons. Because Amaterasu, the Sun, is responsible for the regeneration of nature and thereby the survival of mankind, it is incumbent upon humans to attend to her needs. In Ise, Amaterasu and the divinities present with her are all fed and have their clothes changed and their rooms swept out regularly. And at the appointed time their dwellings are completely rebuilt. That tradition, known as *Shikinen Sengu*, dates back to the year 660. Every twenty years, most recently in 2013, Ise Shrine is disassembled and reconstructed exactly as it was. Reconstruction lasts eight years. Each edifice of the Inner Shrine (*Naiku*), each edifice of the Outer Shrine (*Geku*), the fourteen major auxiliary shrines (*Betsugu*), and the one hundred and nine minor ones are all rebuilt. The material presence there – bridges, porticos, fences, buildings, clothing – is revered precisely because it is perishable. The process of regeneration appears in the grand repertory of rituals. *Shikinen Sengu* is the story of that regeneration, with a new structure always identical to the previous one erected every twenty years. It symbolizes the uninterrupted cycle of life.

In Europe, the cathedrals built to last for all eternity were two hundred years in the making. Here, destruction and reconstruction, which is to say uncertainty and impermanence, are the pillars on which Shinto spirituality rests. In Japan, twenty years represents one cycle in a person's life, and is celebrated as such. They begin disassembling buildings after twelve years, which is the time it takes Jupiter to revolve around the Sun and the Moon to revolve around the Earth. The number 12 represents perfection. Reconstruction takes eight years, 8 being the number that represents creation through movement, incarnation into matter, and abiding eternity.

天照
Amaterasu

The house of Amaterasu is hidden behind four high wooden fences. By peering over them, visitors can glimpse a structure similar to a rice granary with a thatched roof and big wood pillars. The main building is said to house the Sacred Mirror, *Yata no Kagami*, which is in a coffer kept in a repository resembling a tabernacle. The mirror represents the sun reflecting onto the world below and symbolizes wisdom and the ability to understand. It is one of the Three Sacred Treasures of Japan, the two others being the sword, *Kusanagi no Tsurugi*, housed in the Atsuta Shrine and which stands for the virtues of valor, and a jewel, *Yasakani no Magatama*, symbol of benevolence and the ability to learn. Amaterasu gave these three treasures to her grandson Ninigi-no-Mikoto, the great-grandfather of Japan's first emperor, Jimmu Tenno.

We hurried along through the throng, up the steps and through the torii. I was not about to get the ritual wrong. I used a small ladle to pour water onto my hands, first the left, then the right, then ladled more water into my left hand and raised it to my lips. I bowed in front of the torii. At the shrine entrance, I set down a coin, a 50-yen piece with a hole in the middle. I rang the bell to alert the gods to my presence. I bowed twice, breathing in, breathing out, breathing in, breathing out. My lungs filled with the air of the forest and its thousand-year-old trees. I clapped my hands twice. Some pilgrims spread their arms wide, expanding their chests, and clapped loudly. I followed their lead, then bowed once more.

The Emperor is supposed to be the only person allowed beyond the second fence. So who were these people that a priest in a mauve habit and a gold-colored hat had escorted in? Then I saw them advancing towards the third fence! There was even a blond-haired woman in the group! Probably Putin's daughter, someone behind us quipped, and some of the pilgrims chuckled. The priest came to a halt. Putin's daughter came up to him and bowed flawlessly. As she was exiting another family in their Sunday best came in to go through the same ritual. We would later learn that this privilege was reserved for the patrons of Ise Jingu. Any rice or tomato grower, any artisan or farmer who helped finance the reconstruction earned the right to put the Amaterasu label on his products. We walked around the magnificent grounds for hours, bowed to hundreds of kami. Even though we hadn't slept we felt wonderfully serene and regenerated.

In Jin Shin Jyutsu, the energy of the Sun (the seventh depth) becomes the first depth after entering the body through the spleen, which is associated with the astrological sign Cancer (June 22 - July 22). The energetic function of the spleen begins in the big toe and terminates in the heart. It permeates the soul with the energy of the Sun, gives the heart its spark, and sends energy to all the organs in the body. The spleen is coupled with the stomach. Together they constitute the energy of Mother Earth. They are the organs of growth and digestion and form the first depth. Mary Burmeister recommended that we harmonize our spleen and stomach flows daily. In the *Kojiki* we read that the Sun, Amaterasu, ensures the regeneration of our bodies. Jin Shin Jyutsu teaches us to maintain the energy of the Sun in our bodies. One way of doing so is to hold our thumb, which stimulates the spleen and the stomach flows.

That night we moved into an actual room at the guesthouse. They were bare-bone accommodations, but it felt like the height of luxury. Early the following day at dawn, before leaving for Kumano, we would visit another part of the grounds and pay tribute to Amaterasu's younger brother, the Moon.

月
Moon

I am quite moved by the kanji for the Moon.

Tsuki, the Moon, is the younger brother of Amaterasu. The Moon illuminates the night, but without the Sun it wouldn't be much.

Tsuki resides near its parents, Izanagi and Izanami.

Deep in the forest we came upon four identical structures that looked like rice granaries.

Izanami, Izanagi, Tsukiyomi no miya, and Tsukiyomi aramitama no miya.

The legend recounted in the *Kojiki* presents Izanami and Izanagi as the deities responsible for the creation.

In the beginning, the Earth was empty. These two gods were

given the mission of shaping the chaos. They plunged a celestial spear into the ocean. The eight drops of solid ground that dripped down from it formed the Japanese archipelago. Then Izanami and Izanagi engendered numerous kami, mountains, waterfalls, trees, and animals... everything found in nature. After many a misadventure, they created the cycle of life and death. Finally, when Izanagi returned from a stay in the underworld, he purified himself in a bath and begot more kami:

Tsukiyomo, kami of the Moon, who came out of his right eye
Amaterasu, kami of the Sun, who came out of his left eye,
Susanoo, kami of the Storm, who came out of his nose.

I cleansed my hands and my mouth and began bowing. We were the only people there. The Moon does not attract nearly as many visitors as the Sun. As we drew closer to the four buildings, Kyoko pointed out that there was an order to them, and that the Moon had two houses, one for its body, one for its soul. There was an order in which to bow, too.

I bowed to Tsukiyomi no miya, the Moon.

I bowed to Tsukiyomi aramitama no miya, the soul of the Moon.

I bowed to Azanagi, the father.

I bowed to Azanami, the mother.

The father was on one side of the body of the Moon, and the soul of the Moon on the other.

In Jin Shin Jyutsu, the Moon is the planet of the sixth depth, which is the mirror of the universe. The history of mankind is manifest in the main central vertical energy, the spine, and travels up the back and down the front of the body; as above, so below; as below, so above. The diaphragm, with its ascending energy, and the umbilicus, with its descending energy, are associated with the sixth depth. You can hold the palm of your hand to activate the energy of the main central.

You do not have to be fluent in Japanese or know the ways of Shinto worship to go on this pilgrimage and honor the gods. The ritual is extremely simple: you press your palms together and you bow.

By the time we left Ise Jingu, I was convinced that the secrets of the universe were somehow revealed there: in the number of temples, in their location, and in the symbolic meaning of objects and rituals. Murai Sensi had led me to Ise, but not to bow before some old text of his that would attest to his work. In the library in Ise, I had felt his presence leaning over old Shinto texts, working tirelessly. He had developed an interest in each of the deities in Ise and studied their roles. He had studied the paths that led from the Outer Shrine to the Inner Shrine. He had counted the torii, sketched the bridges, and gently touched the thousand-year-old trees. He had dreamed the 26 points of energy, the trinity flow, the mediator and supervisor flows. And there in Ise, Jiro Murai, master among masters, had laughed and whispered in my ear: "What I discovered, you can discover, too."

Jin Shin Jyutsu Is.

Arigato, Murai Sensei
Paris, June 18, 2018

Getting to Know (Help) Myself

(Excerpts from Book I of *Introducing Jin Shin Jyutsu Is*, by Mary Burmeister. Jin Shin Jyutsu, Inc., Scottsdale, Arizona, 1994)

Basic Daily Practices

The following three sequences are for general daily supply of energy by simply utilizing combinations of the 26 "keys" for unlocking the "safety energy locks" located on the "monitor" or "supervisor" energy pattern.

1. For General Energy Revitalizing

A. For the RIGHT Side of the Body:

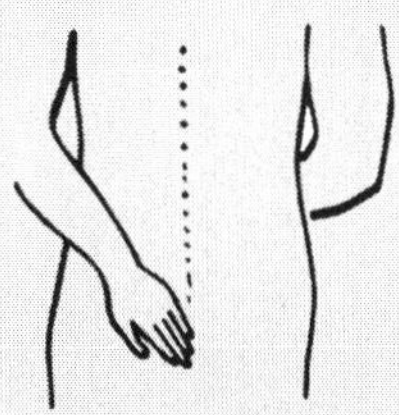

(1) Place left hand (palm side or back of hand, whichever is most comfortable) at base of spine (coccyx).

(2) Place right hand on RIGHT medial (inner) side of ankle bone (between inner side ankle bone and inner side heel).

If the above position is uncomfortable, place right fingers on RIGHT medial (inner) side of knee, or place right fingers on the pubic bone. No straining is necessary to unlock any of the 26 "safety energy locks." There are no "should's" or "have to's." Just comfortably apply sequence. It is simply "Getting to KNOW (Help) MYSELF."

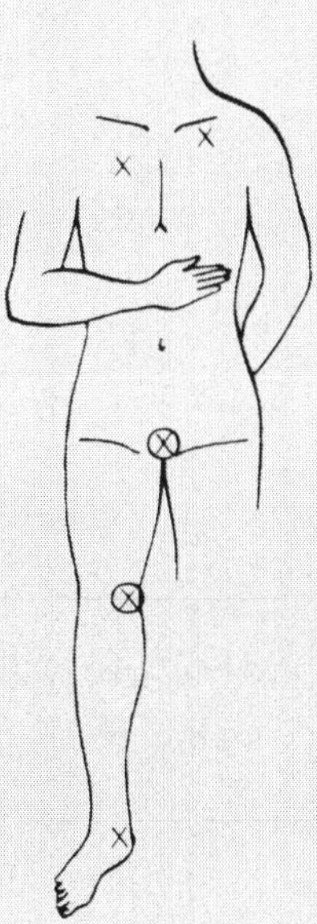

(3) Replace right hand only to base of center of LEFT front rib cage.

(4) Replace left hand only to center of RIGHT third rib from right clavicle (collar bone), just above right breast area.

(5) Replace left hand only to center of LEFT clavicle (collar bone) between clavicle and first rib.

b. For the LEFT Side of the Body:

The sequence for the LEFT side of the body is in reverse of the RIGHT side. As time permits, both right and left sequences may be applied. However, if time does not permit applying to both sides of the body, only the more tense side need be applied. Simply allot time available to the 5 steps. When your "allotted" time is up, or when you become aware of the rhythm of the universe in each step, simply move on to the next step. There are no rigid rules. Simply adjust the sequence to your own convenience and comfort. If, for instance, a "step" feels most revitalizing to you, just get into the habit, in your art of LIVING, of utilizing that step as your own "special quickie" revitalizing exercise. The art of LIVING is simple. You are the "artist."

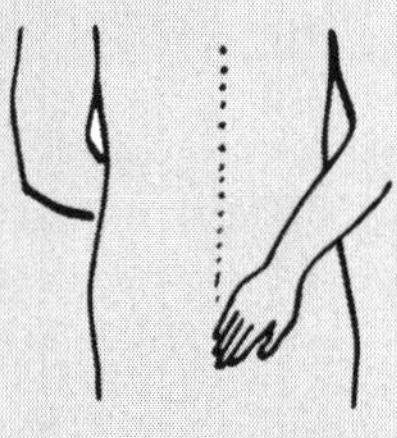

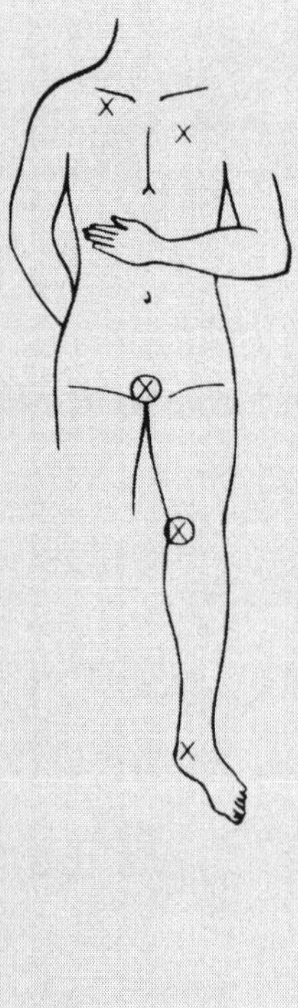

(1) Place right hand (palm side or back of hand, whichever is most comfortable) at base of spine (coccyx).

(2) Place left hand on LEFT medial ankle bone (between inner side ankle bone and heel).

NOTE: If this position is uncomfortable, place fingers on the LEFT medial (inner) side of knee, or place your left fingers on the pubic bone. No straining is necessary to unlock any of the 26 "safety energy locks." Remember, there are no "should's" or "have to's." Simply hold each position in your most comfortable way.

(3) Replace left hand only to base of center of RIGHT front rib cage. Right hand is still at the base of the spine (coccyx).

(4) Replace right hand only to center of LEFT third rib from LEFT clavicle (collar bone), right above LEFT breast area.

(5) Replace right hand only to center of RIGHT clavicle (collar bone) between clavicle and first rib.

NOTE: Helps to revitalize energy, "refuel."

2. For General Daily Energy Revitalizing of ANTERIOR DESCENDING Energy

(Down the Front of the Body)

A. For the RIGHT side of the Body:

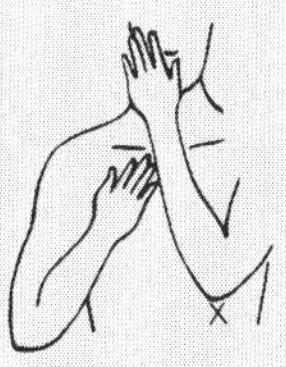

(1) Place left finger or fingers on base of RIGHT cheek bone.

(2) Place right finger or fingers at center of RIGHT clavicle (collar bone).

(3) Place right finger or fingers only to base of center of LEFT front rib cage.

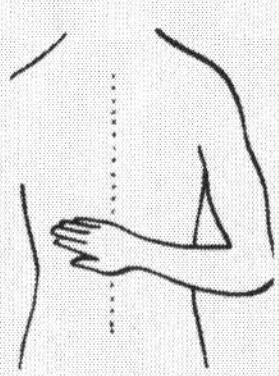

(4) Place right finger or fingers only to LEFT small of back (above LEFT waist at base of LEFT back rib cage).

NOTE:
Always know that any step you are not able to reach comfortably you can skip and go on to the next step you are able to reach without strain. You may not be able to feel the rhythm of the universe at first, but with patience you can soon begin to feel the pulsation, or feel a relaxation in the "connection."

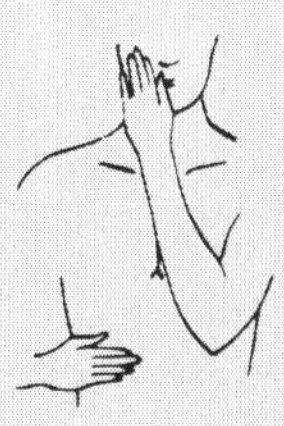

(5) Replace the right finger or fingers only to base of center of RIGHT front rib cage.

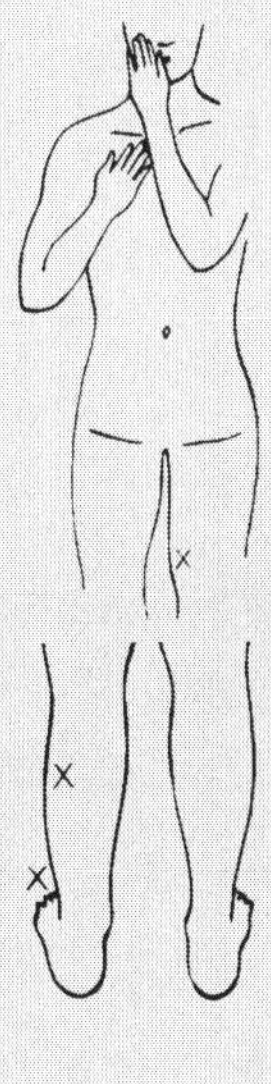

(6) Replace right finger or fingers only to medial (inner) side of LEFT thigh about 3" above LEFT knee.

(7) Replace right finger or fingers only halfway down calf about midway, between lateral (outer) side of knee and ankle, off the LEFT shin bone.

(8) Replace right finger or fingers only to LEFT middle toe (sandwich middle toe with a finger and thumb).

NOTE:
Left finger or fingers have been on the base of RIGHT cheek bone throughout this sequence, and only the right finger or fingers have been moved.

Aids in releasing tensions causing head, breathing, digestive discomforts and bloating, as well as weight problems.

A. For the LEFT side of the Body:

NOTE: The sequence for the LEFT side of the body is in reverse of the RIGHT side. As time permits, both the right and left sequences may be applied. However, if time does not permit, or there is no need to apply both the left and right sequences, only the side more tense need be applied. Simply allot available time to the 8 steps, moving from one step to the next according to time allotted, or when the rhythm of the universe is felt. Again, only those steps particularly comfortable for you need be applied, as this may be just the "modified" or "individualized" sequence needed for your body at that time.

The 26 "safety energy locks" are our own "individualized" Art of LIVING, the Getting to KNOW (Help) MYSELF.

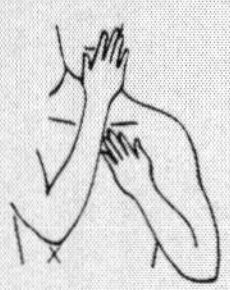

(1) Place right finger or fingers on base of LEFT cheek bone.

(2) Place left finger or fingers at center of LEFT clavicle (collar bone).

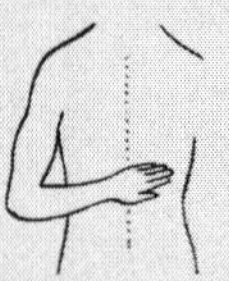

(3) Replace left finger or fingers only to base of center of RIGHT front rib cage.

(4) Replace left finger or fingers only to RIGHT small of back (above RIGHT waist at base of RIGHT back rib cage).

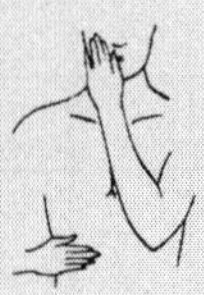

(5) Replace left finger or fingers only to base of center of LEFT front rib cage.

(6) Replace left finger or fingers only to medial (inner) side of RIGHT thigh about 3" above RIGHT knee.

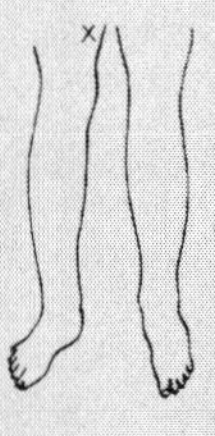

(7) Replace left finger or fingers only to halfway down calf, about midway between lateral (outer) side of knee and ankle, off RIGHT shin bone.

(8) Replace left finger or fingers only to RIGHT middle toe (just sandwich middle toe with a finger and thumb).

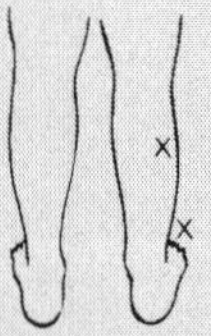

NOTE:
Aids in releasing tensions causing head, breathing, digestive discomforts. (Steps (1) and (6) may be used to aid in releasing tensions causing abdominal, bloating, and weight discomforts.)

3. For General Daily "Individualized" Body Energy Revitalizing of POSTERIOR DESCENDING (Down the Back of the Body) Energy:

a. For the RIGHT side of the Body:

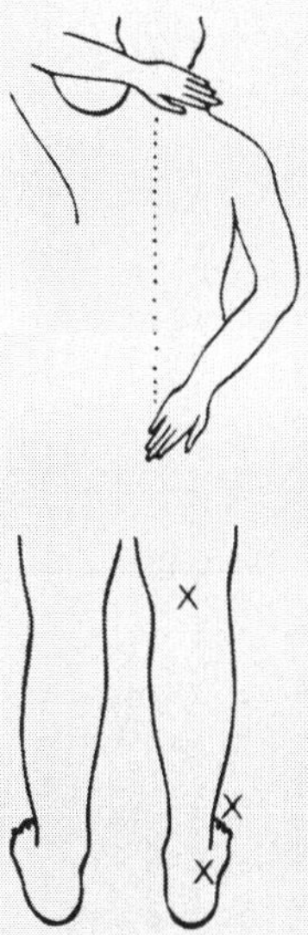

(1) Place left finger or fingers on RIGHT side of cervicals (on neck between ear and spine).

(2) Place right hand (back of hand or palm side) at base of spine (coccyx).

Replace right finger or fingers only to center of back of RIGHT knee.

(4) Replace right finger or fingers only to RIGHT lateral (outer) side ankle below RIGHT ankle bone.

(5) Replace right finger or fingers only to RIGHT little toe (sandwich little toe with thumb and a finger).

NOTE:
Aids in releasing tensions causing head, back, elimination and leg discomforts.

Simply – Getting to KNOW (Help) MYSELF

b. For the LEFT Side of the Body:

NOTE:
The sequence for the LEFT side of body is in reverse of the RIGHT side. As time permits, both the right and left sequences may be applied. However, if time does not permit, or there is no need to apply to both the left and right sides of the body, only the side that is more tense need be applied. Simply allot the available time to the 5 steps, moving from one "safety energy lock" to the next for the time allotted, or when the rhythm of the universe is felt. Again, if a "safety energy lock" is uncomfortable to reach, skip it and go on to the next comfortable step, knowing that it is "individualized" by you for you.

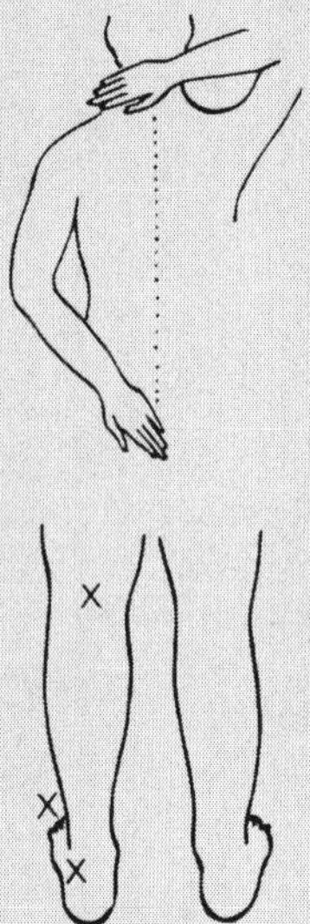

(1) Place right finger or fingers on LEFT side of cervicals (on neck between ear and spine).

(2) Place left hand (back of hand or palm side) at base of spine (coccyx).

(3) Replace left finger or fingers only to center of back of LEFT knee.

(4) Replace left finger or fingers only to LEFT lateral (outer side) ankle below LEFT ankle bone.

(5) Replace left finger or fingers only to LEFT little toe (sandwich little toe with thumb and a finger).

NOTE:
Aids in releasing tensions causing head, back, elimination, leg discomforts.

JIN SHIN JYUTSU is our inheritance. All we need is desire for awareness. It is Getting to KNOW (Help) MYSELF.

The three sequences outlined above are for special daily maintenance to be in complete harmony mentally, emotionally, digestively, and physically.

Simply – Getting to KNOW (Help) MYSELF

Notes

1. Mieko Macé, *Médecins et médecine dans l'histoire du Japon*. Les Belles Lettres, 2013, p. 238.
2. Pierre Vinclair, *Kojiki*. Le Corridor bleu, 2011, p. 185.
3. Mary Burmeister, *Introducing Jin Shin Jyutsu Is, Book I*. Jin Shin Jyutsu, Inc, Scottsdale, Arizona, 1994.
4. *Haïku. Anthologie du poème court japonais*, Edited and translated by Corinne Atlan and Zéno Bianu. Gallimard, 2002, p. 14.
5. Mary Burmeister, as cited by instructors in workshops.
6. 加藤春樹、『仁神術』、たにぐち書店、Jin Shin Jyutsu, Taniguchi, 2002.
7. Matthias Roth, *Tisser. Module 2*, workshop workbook.
8. Mary Burmeister, as cited by instructors in workshops.
9. Pierre Vinclair, op. cit (note 2), p. 149.
10. Mary Burmeister, *Text 1*, Jin Shin Jyutsu. Inc., Scottsdale, Arizona, 1997, p. 13.
11. Ibid.
12. *Basho, Seigneur ermite: L'Intégrale des haïkus*, édition bilingue. La Table ronde, 2012. ; See note 14 regarding quotations of Basho throughout this book.
13. Pierre Vinclair, op. cit. (note 2), p. 101.
14. Matsuo Basho, *Le Chemin étroit vers les contrées du Nord*, translated by Nicolas Bouvier. Héros-Limite, 2006. Throughout this book, Basho's haiku will henceforth be cited (without page or haiku numbers for reasons of fre quency) according to the editions referenced in notes 12 and 14, as well as: *A Haiku Garden, The Four Seasons in Poems and Prints*, edited by Stephen Addiss. Weatherhill, 1996; and *Haïku. Anthologie du poème court japonais*, op. cit. (note 4).
15. Haruki Murakami, *Kafka sur le rivage*, translated by Corinne Atlan. Belfond, 2006, p. 69.

16. Hiraide Takashi, *Le Chat qui venait du ciel,* translated by Elisabeth Suetsugu. Éditions Philippe Picquier, 2017.
17. Terada Torahiko, *L'Esprit du haïku,* translated by Olivier Birmann and Hiroki Toura. Éditions Philippe Picquier, 2016, p. 48.
18. Roland Barthes, *L'Empire des signes*. Seuil, 2015, p. 106.
19. Véronique Le Normand and Natali Fortier, *J'aime*. Albin Michel, 2004; Minne and Natali Fortier, *I Love*. Kane Miller Books, 2005.
20. Haruki Murakami, op. cit. (note 15), p. 69.
21. Ibid., p. 52.
22. Junichiro Tanizaki, *Éloge de l'ombre,* translated by René Sieffert. Verdier, 2011, p. 47.
23. Lafcadio Hearn, *Le Japon, translated* by Marc Logé and Joseph de Smet. Collection Mille pages, Mercure de France, 1921, p. 66.
24. Tzolkin Application to the Human Body. A theory developed by Aaron Driver.
25. Matsuo Basho, op. cit. (note 14), p. 61.
26. Pierre Vinclair, op. cit. (note 2), p. 56.
27. Luis Frois, *Européens et Japonais. Traité des contradictions et différences,* translated by Xavier de Castro. Chandeigne, 1998, p. 73.
28. Junichiro Tanizaki, op. cit. (note 22), p. 20.
29. Xavier de Castro, *La Découverte du Japon*, 1543-1552; Chandeigne (18 mai 2017).
30. Mieko Macé, op. cit. (note 1), p. 78.
31. David Mitchell, *Les Mille Automnes de Jacob de Zoet*. L'Olivier, 2012.
32. Patrick Deville, *La Peste et le Choléra*. Seuil, 2012.
33. Haruki Kato, *Jin Shin Jyutsu*. Taniguchi, 2002. Selected quotations translated by Kyoko Watanabe.
34. Luis Frois, op. cit. (note 27), p. 63 (articles 3 et 5), p. 64 (article 9), p. 65 (article 18).
35. Cited in: Anne Millerand, "La modernisation de la

médecine japonaise d'Edo à Meiji. Rupture ou continuité." PhD Dissertation, 2011, p. 172.

36. Ibid.
37. Mieko Macé, op. cit. (note 1), p. 22.
38. Jean Herbert, *Aux sources du Japon*, le shintô. Albin Michel, 1964, chapitre ii.
39. Akira Mizubayashi, *Une langue venue d'ailleurs*. Gallimard, 2011, p. 87.
40. Luis Frois, op. cit. (note 27), p. 47 (article 2).
41. Louis Frédéric, *Fêtes et traditions au pays du Soleil levan*t. Société Continentale d'Éditions modernes illustrées, 1970.
42. Haïku, op. cit. (note 4), p. 38.
43. Didier Decoin, *Le Bureau des jardins et des étangs*. Stock, 2016.
44. Haïku, op. cit. (note 4), p. 92.
45. Jean Herbert, *Le Japon: croyances et rites*. Dervy, 2015, p. 120.
46. Haruki Murakami, *Après le tremblement de terre*. 10/18,2002.
47. Haïku, op. cit. (note 4), p. 122.
48. Ibid., p. 143.
49. Ibid., p. 142.
50. Junichirô Tanizaki, *Le Chat, son maître et ses deux maîtresses*, translated by Cécile Sakai. Folio, 2017.
51. Akira Mizubayashi, *Mélodie*. Gallimard, 2013, p. 328.
52. Haïku, op. cit. (note 4), p. 176.
53. Hosai, *Dans la boîte à clous tous les clous sont tordus*. Moundarren, 2000.
54. Bertrand Petit, Keiko Yokoyama, *L'Adieu du samouraï*. Éditions Alternatives, 2003, p. 46.
55. Kyuya Fukada, *One Hundred Mountains of Japan*, translated by Martin Hood. University of Hawaii Press, 2014.
56. Erri de Luca, *Sur la trace de Nives*, translated by Danièle Valin. Folio, 2013.
57. Mary Burmeister, op. cit. (note 3), p. 1.
58. Alice Burmeister and Tom Monte, *The Touch of Healing:*

Energizing Body, Mind, and Spirit with the Art of Jin Shin Jyutsu. Bantam Books, 1997, p. 15.

59. Alice Burmeister and Tom Monte, op. cit. (note 58), p. 27.
60. Mary Burmeister, op. cit. (note 3), p. 1.
61. Carl Gustav Jung, *Psychologie et orientalisme,* translated by Paul Kessler, Josette Rigal and Rainer Rochlitz. Albin Michel, 1985, p. 195.
62. Shichiro Fukazawa, *Narayama,* translated by Bernard Frank. Gallimard, 1980.
63. Sylvain Guintard-Kuban, *Ascèse de l'eau*. www.shugendo.fr.
64. Luis Frois, op. cit. (note 27), p. 57 (article 41).
65. Michel Odoul, *Le Shiatsu*. PUF, Que sais-je ?, no 4079, 2017, p. 25.
66. Mary Burmeister, *Text I,* op. cit. (note 10), p. 1.
67. Luis Frois, op. cit. (note 27), p. 47 (article 7).
68. Durian Sukegawa, *Les délices de Tokyo*. Le Livre de Poche, 2017. Film by Naomi Kawase (2015).
69. Haruki Kato, op. cit. (note 33).
70. Ibid.
71. Mary Burmeister, op. cit. (note 3), p. 2.
72. Véronique Le Normand and Natali Fortier, op. cit. (note 19), Albin Michel, 2003.
73. Luis Frois, op. cit. (note 27), p. 72 (article 17).
74. Paul Claudel, "À travers les villes en flamme." In: *Ebisu*, no 21, 1999. Le Japon de séismes, 1999, p. 35-47.
75. Ibid.
76. Source: Wikipédia, article "Bombardement de Tokyo."
77. Blaise Pascal, *Pensées*, 1670. Le Livre de poche, 2000, #430.
78. Takashi Nagai, *Une lumière dans Nagasaki*, anthologie. La Nouvelle Cité, 2006.
79. François Laplantine, *Le Japon ou le Sens des extrêmes*. Pocket, 2017, p. 19.
80. Yasunari Kawabata, *Chronique d'Asakusa*, translated by Suzanne Rosset. Le Livre de poche, 1992.

81. Based on *"What Mary says, ..."* by Mary Burmeister and freely interpreted by the author.
82. Cited in: Tanaka Yuko and Cadou Catherine. "Le monde comme représentation symbolique. Le Japon de l'époque d'Edo et l'univers du mitate." In: *Annales. Histoire, Sciences Sociales*. 50e année, N. 2, 1995. p. 259-281.
83. Yoko Tawada, *Journal des jours tremblants après Fukushima, précédé de Leçons de poétique*, translated from German by Bernard Banoun and from Japanese by Cécile Sakai. Verdier, 2012, p. 91-93.
84. Toson Shimazaki, *La Transgression*, translated by Suzanne Rosset. You-Feng, 1999.
85. Mary Burmeister, op. cit. (note 3), p. 6.
86. Natsume Soseki, *Je suis un chat*, translated by Jean Cholley. Gallimard, 1978, p. 23.
87. Sei Shonagon, *Les Notes de l'oreiller*, translated by Kuni Matsuo and Steinibler-Oberlin. Stock, 1990, p. 21.

Bibliography

- *Kojiki*, Pierre Vinclair. Le Corridor bleu, 2011.
- *Haïku. Anthologie du poème court japonais*, edited and translated by Corinne Atlan and Zéno Bianu. Gallimard, 2002.
- *Le Sanctuaire d'Ise. Récit de la 62e reconstruction.* Jean-Sébastein Cluzel, Masatsugu Nishida. Mardaga, 2015.
- Roland Barthes, *L'Empire des signes*. Seuil, 2015.
- Matsuo Basho, *Le Chemin étroit vers les contrées du Nord*, translated by Nicolas Bouvier. Héros-Limite, 2006.
- Nicolas Bouvier, *Chronique japonaise*. Payot, 1989.
- Mary Burmeister, *Introducing Jin Shin Jyutsu Is, Book I. Jin Shin Jyutsu*. Inc., Scottsdale, Arizona, 1994.
- Alice Burmeister and Tom Monte, *The Touch of Healing: Energizing Body, Mind, and Spirit with the Art of Jin Shin Jyutsu*. Bantam Books, 1997.
- Kamo no Chomei, *Notes de ma cabane de moine*, translated by Révérend Père Sauveur Candau. Le Bruit du temps, 2010.
- Louis Frédéric, *Fêtes et traditions au pays du Soleil levant*. Société continentale d'éditions modernes, 1970.
- Luis Frois, *Européens et Japonais. Traité des contradictions et differences*, translated by Xavier de Castro. Chandeigne, 1998.
- Lafcadio Hearn, *Le Japon*. Mercure de France, 1921.
- Jean Herbert, *Le Japon : croyances et rites*. Dervy, 2015.
- Gertrud Hirshi, *Les Mudras. Le yoga au bout des doigts*. Le Courrier du livre, 1998.
- 加藤春樹、『仁神術』、たにぐち書店、2002年。この本からの引用はすべて 渡辺響子が口頭で翻訳した。(Haruki Kato, *Jin Shin Jyutsu*. édition Taniguchi, 2002).
- Mieko Macé, *Médecins et médecine dans l'histoire du Japon*. Les Belles Lettres, 2013.
- René Sieffert, *La Littérature japonaise*. Publications orientalistes de France, 2000.
- Junichiro Tanizaki, *Éloge de l'ombre*. Verdier, 2011.

My Favorite Films

Clint Eastwood (1930-)
Letters from Iwo Jima, 2006

Shoshei Imamura (1926-2006)
The Eel, 1997

Naomi Kawase (1969-)
Sweet Bean, 2015

Keisuke Kinoshita (1912-1998)
The Ballad of Narayama, 1983
The Children of Nagasaki, 1983
Twenty-Four Eyes, 1954

Hirokazu Kore-Eda (1962-)
After the Storm, 2016
Still Walking, 2008

Akira Kurosawa (1910-1998)
Drunken Angel, 1948
Rashomon, 1950
Red Beard, 1965
Ran, 1985

Hayao Miyazaki (1941-)
The Wind Rises, 2013
My Neighbor Totoro, 1988

Kenji Mizoguchi (1898-1956)
Tales of Ugetsu,1953
The Life of Oharu, 1952

Nagisa Oshima (1932-2013)
Empire of Passion, 1978
In the Realm of the Senses, 1976
Boy, 1969

Yasujiro Ozu (1903-1963)
Tokyo Chorus, 1931
There Was a Father, 1942
Late Spring, 1949
Tokyo Story, 1953

Alain Resnais (1922-2014)
Hiroshima mon amour, 1959

Martin Scorcese (1942-)
Silence, 2016

Kaneto Shindo (1912-2012)
The Naked Island, 1960

Yojiro Takita (1955-)
Departures, 2006

Acknowledgments

My sincere thanks to all the Japanese people mentioned in this book for so generously making themselves available, for their extreme kindness, and their amused curiosity. I am grateful to all those with whom I crossed paths and who, with a simple word or the title of a book or film, opened new horizons for me.

My special thanks to Sadaki Kato, Alexandre Leroi-Cortot, Michèle and Akira Mizubayashi, Misako Nemoto, and Inger Van Dobben.

Special thanks, too, to Danielle Blanc, "the messenger," Thierry Magnier, "the courier," and Anne-Sylvie Bameule, my editor.

I would also like to thank David Burmeister and Nathalie Max for the use of JSJ, Inc. materials.

I will never be able to thank Kyoko Watanabe enough for sharing her country with me, forever to love.

Also Available from UWSP

- *November Rose: A Speech on Death* by Kathrin Stengel (2008 Independent Publisher Book Award)
- *November-Rose: Eine Rede über den Tod* by Kathrin Stengel
- *Philosophical Fragments of a Contemporary Life* by Julien David
- *17 Vorurteile, die wir Deutschen gegen Amerika und die Amerikaner haben und die so nicht ganz stimmen können* by Misha Waiman
- *The DNA of Prejudice: On the One and the Many* by Michael Eskin (2010 Next Generation Indie Book Award for Social Change)
- *Descartes' Devil: Three Meditations* by Durs Grünbein
- *Fatal Numbers: Why Count on Chance* by Hans Magnus Enzensberger
- *The Vocation of Poetry by Durs Grünbein* (2011 Independent Publisher Book Award for Poetry)
- *The Waiting Game: An Essay on the Gift of Time* by Andrea Köhler (out of print)
- *Mortal Diamond: Poems* by Durs Grünbein
- *Yoga for the Mind: A New Ethic for Thinking and Being & Meridians of Thought* by Michael Eskin and Kathrin Stengel (2014 Living Now Book Award)
- *The Wisdom of Parenthood: An Essay* by Michael Eskin
- *Health is in Your Hands: Jin Shin Jyutsu—Practicing the Art of Self-Healing (With 51 Flash Cards for the Hands-On Practice of Jin Shin Jyutsu)* by Waltraud Riegger-Krause (2015 Living Now Book Award for Healing Arts)
- *A Moment More Sublime: A Novel* by Stephen Grant (2015 Independent Publisher Book Award for Contemporary Fiction)
- *High on Low: Harnessing the Power of Unhappiness* by Wilhelm Schmid (2015 Living Now Book Award for Personal Growth and 2015 Independent Publisher Book Award for Self-Help)

- *Become a Message: Poems* by Lajos Walder (2016 Benjamin Franklin Book Award for Poetry)
- *What We Gain As We Grow Older: On Gelassenheit* by Wilhelm Schmid
- *On Dialogic Speech* by L. P. Yakubinsky
- *Passing Time: An Essay on Waiting* by Andrea Köhler
- *In Praise of Weakness* by Alexandre Jollien
- *Vase of Pompeii: A Play* by Lajos Walder
- *Below Zero: A Play* by Lajos Walder
- *Tyrtaeus: A Tragedy* by Lajos Walder
- *The Complete Plays of Lajos Walder* by Lajos Walder
- *Homo Conscius: A Novel* by Timothy Balding
- *Spanish Light: A Novel* by Stephen Grant
- *The Man Who Couldn't Stop Thinking: A Novel* by Timothy Balding
- *Potentially Harmless: A Philosopher's Manhattan* by Kathrin Stengel (forthcoming)
- *The Impostors: A Novel* by Timothy Balding
- *The Complete Poetry of Lajos Walder: A Bilingual Edition* by Lajos Walder
- *Összes Versei* by Vándor Lajos
- *Of Parents and Children: Tools for Nurturing a Lifelong Relationship* by Jorge and Demián Bucay
- *The Zucchini Conspiracy: A Novel of Alternative Facts* by Timothy Balding

Of Related Interest from UWSP

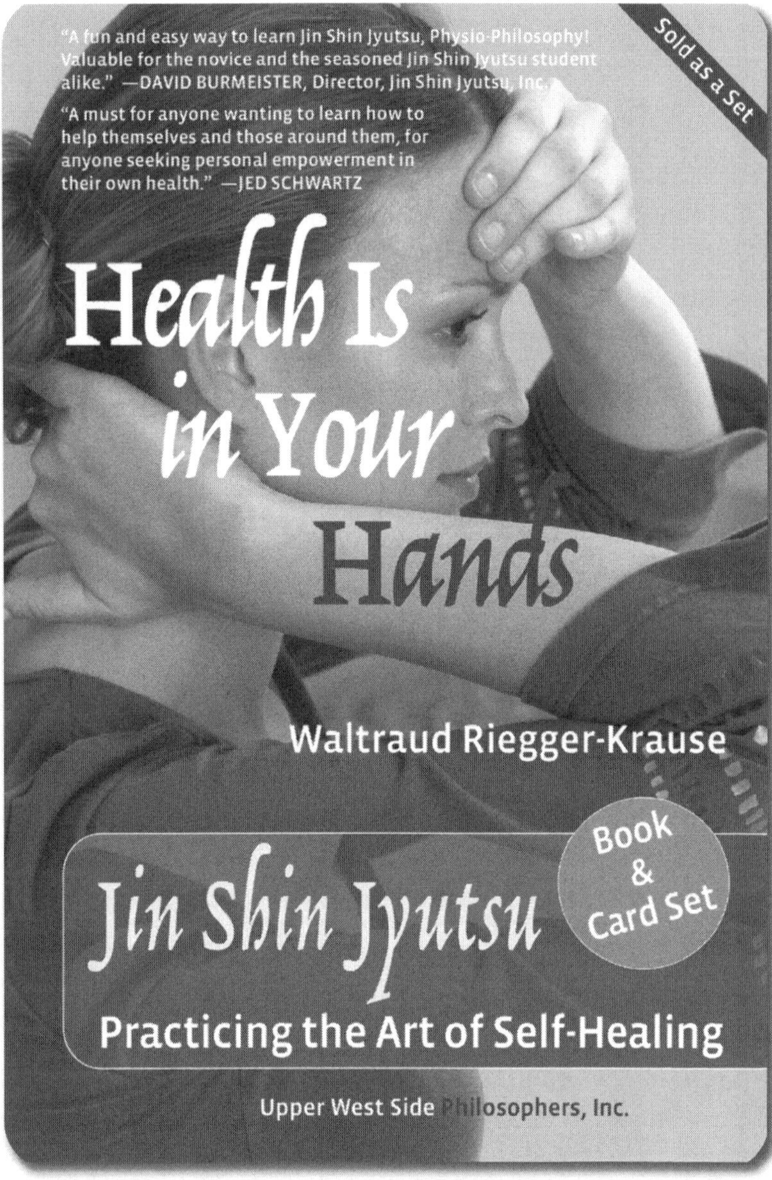

ISBN: 978-1-935830-23-8 (book & card set)
ISBN: 978-1-935830-24-5 (e-book & e-card set)

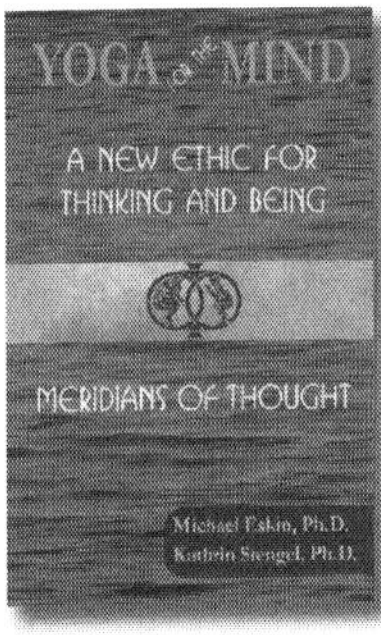

Yoga for the Mind: A New Ethic for Thinking and Being & Meridians of Thought by Michael Eskin & Kathrin Stengel
ISBN: 978-1-935830-09-2 (pbk)
ISBN: 978-1-935830-21-4 (ebook)

The Wisdom of Parenthood: An Essay
by Michael Eskin
ISBN: 978-1-935830-25-2 (pbk)
ISBN: 978-1-935830-26-9 (ebook)

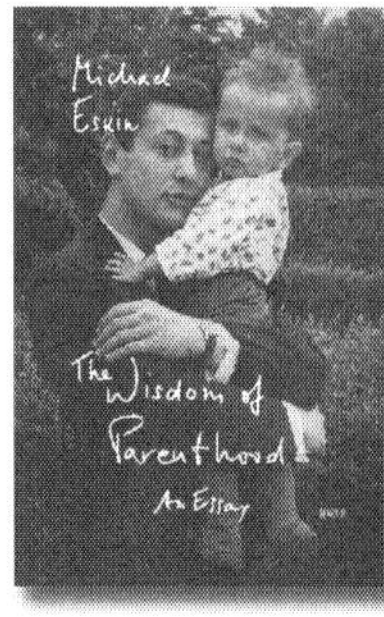

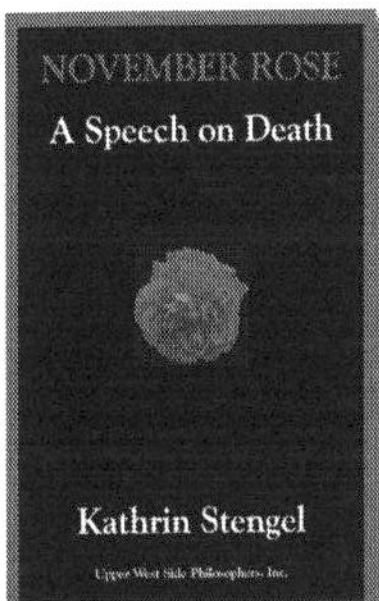

November Rose: A Speech on Death
by Kathrin Stengel
ISBN: 978-1-935830-22-1 (pbk)
ISBN: 978-1-935830-12-2 (ebook)

High on Low: Harnessing the Power of Unhappiness by Wilhelm Schmid
ISBN: 978-1-935830-28-3 (pbk)
ISBN: 978-1-935830-27-6 (ebook)

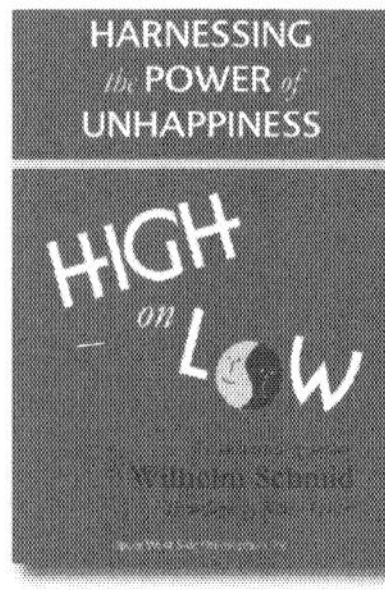

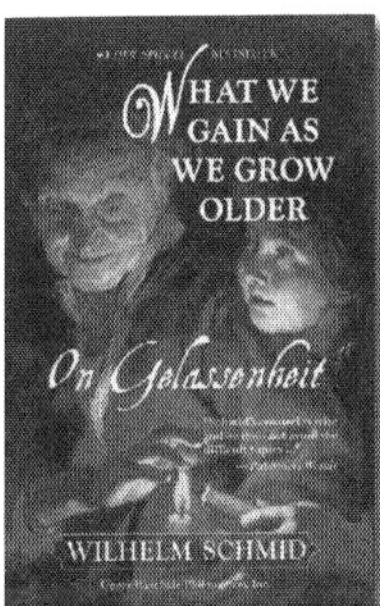

What We Gain as We Grow Older: On Gelassenheit by Wilhelm Schmid
ISBN: 978-1-935830-31-3 (pbk)
ISBN: 978-1-935830-24-5 (ebook)

In Praise of Weakness
by Alexandre Jollien
ISBN: 978-1-935830-42-9 (pbk)
ISBN: 978-1-935830-43-6 (ebook)

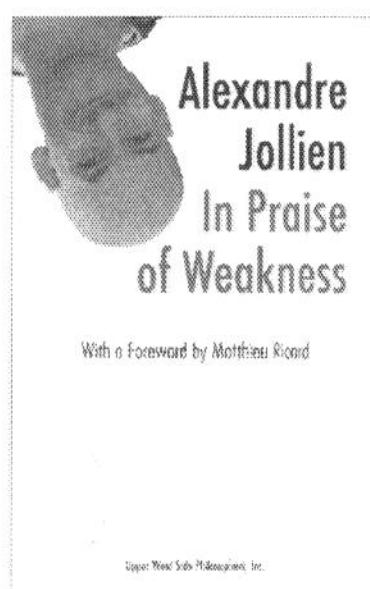

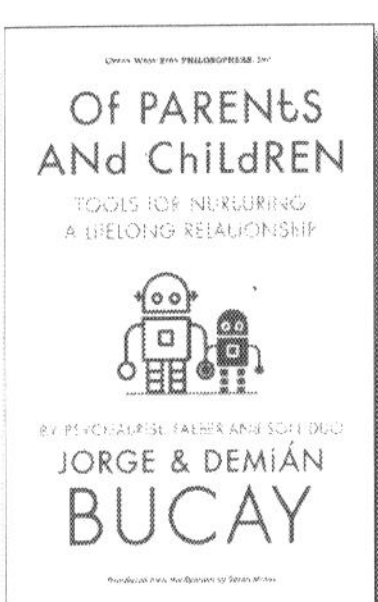

Of Parents and Children: Tools for Nurturing a LIfelong Relationship
by Joge & Demián Bucay
ISBN: 978-1-935830-61-0 (pbk)
ISBN: 978-1-935830-64-1 (ebook)

Passing Time: An Essay on Waiting
by Andrea Köhler
ISBN: 978-1-935830-48-1 (pbk)
ISBN: 978-1-935830-49-8 (ebook)

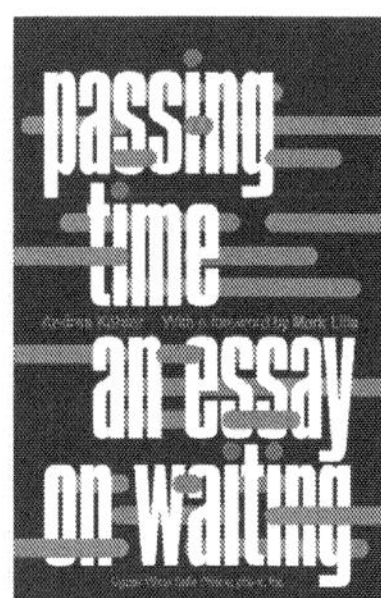

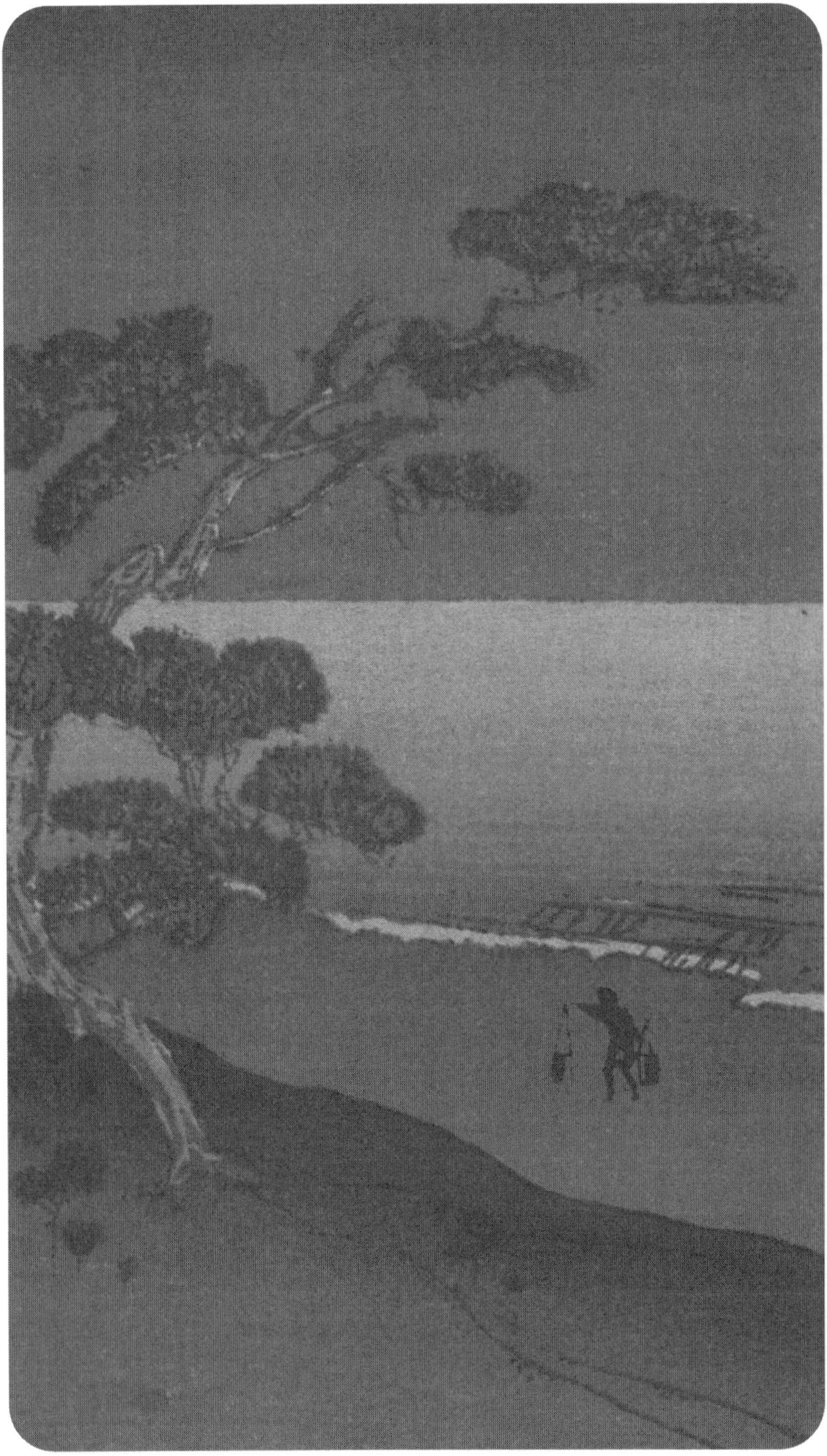

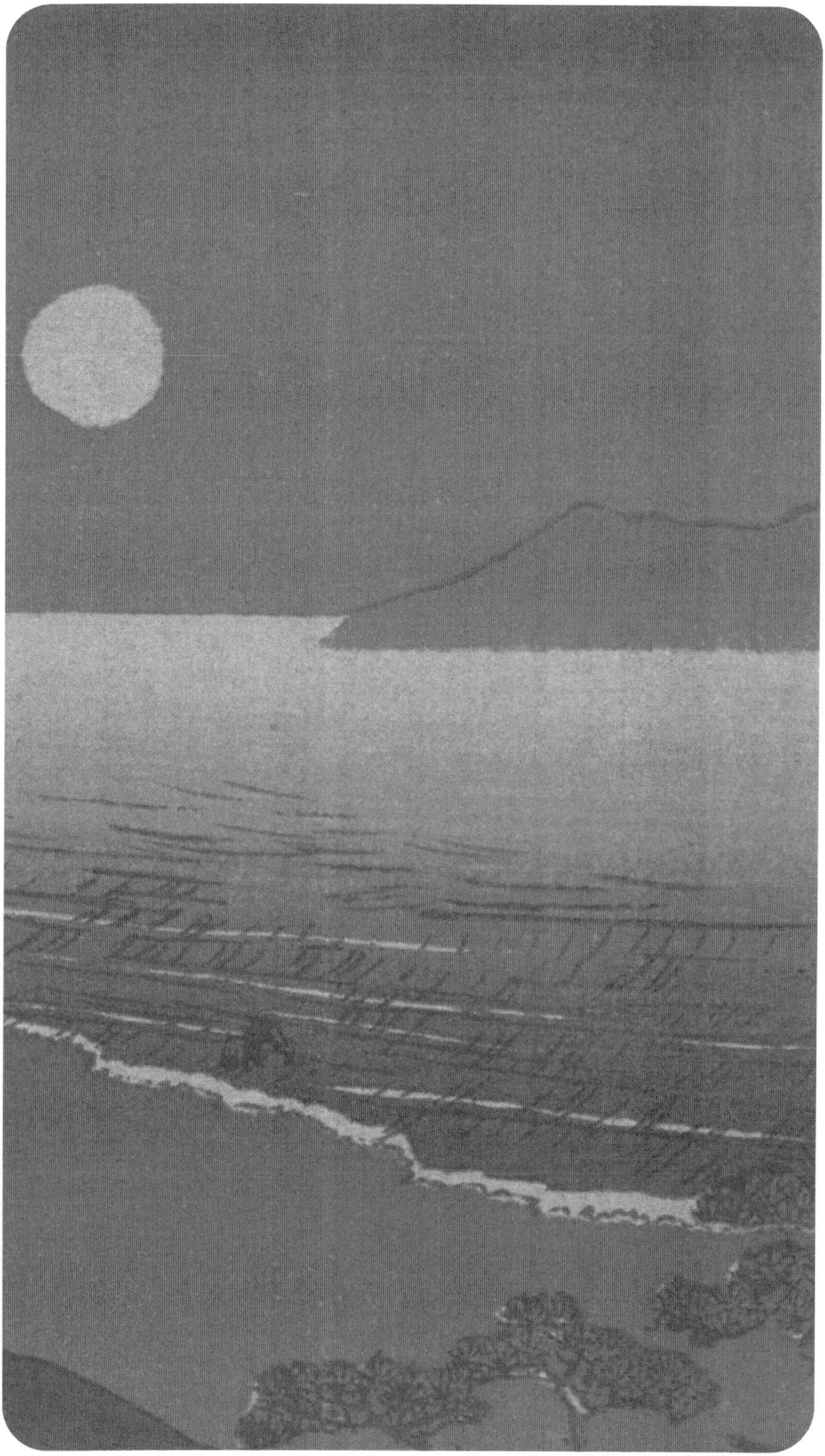

Made in the USA
Middletown, DE
01 April 2022

63430231R00135